Six Steps to **Effective Management**

Managing the Business of Health Care

For Baillière Tindall:

Senior Commissioning Editor: Jacqueline Curthoys
Project Development Editor: Karen Gilmour
Project Manager: Jane Dingwall
Design Direction: George Ajayi

Managing the Business of Health Care

Edited by

Julie Hyde BA(Hons) RGN RCNT RNT CertEd(FE) CertHSM FRSH
MIHM MIMgt MILT
Education, Policy and Management Consultant, UK

Frances E Cooper MPhil RGN DipNurs(Lond) RNT
CertEd DipHealthStudRes
Formerly Director of Nursing and Quality, Royal Wolverhampton Hospitals
NHS Trust, UK

Foreword by

Sir Alan Langlands
Principal and Vice Chancellor, University of Dundee, UK

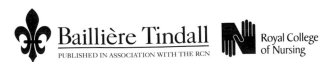

EDINBURGH   LONDON   NEW YORK   PHILADELPHIA   ST LOUIS   SYDNEY   TORONTO   2001

Baillière Tindall
An imprint of Harcourt Publishers Limited

© Harcourt Publishers Limited 2001

✤ is a registered trademark of Harcourt Publishers Limited

The right of Julie Hyde and Frances Cooper to be identified as editors of this work has been asserted by them in accordance with the Copyright, Designs and Patents Act 1988

First published 2001

ISBN 0 7020 2440 6

British Library Cataloguing in Publication Data
A catalogue record for this book is available from the British Library

Library of Congress Cataloging in Publication Data
A catalog record for this book is available from the Library of Congress

Note
Medical knowledge is constantly changing. As new information becomes available, changes in treatment, procedures, equipment and the use of drugs become necessary. The editors, contributors and the publishers have taken care to ensure that the information given in this text is accurate and up to date. However, readers are strongly advised to confirm that the information, especially with regard to drug usage, complies with the latest legislation and standards of practice.

The publisher's policy is to use paper manufactured from sustainable forests

Printed in China

Six Steps to Effective Management series

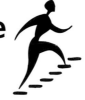

Series Editor: *Ann Young*

Managing the Business of Health Care
Edited by Julie Hyde and Frances Cooper

Managing Diversity and Inequality in Health Care
Edited by Carol Baxter

Managing and Implementing Decisions in Health Care
Edited by Ann Young and Mary Cooke

Managing and Leading Innovation in Health Care
Edited by Elizabeth Howkins and Cynthia Thornton

Managing Communication in Health Care
Edited by Mark Darley

Managing and Supporting People in Health Care
Edited by Margaret Buttigieg and Surrinder Kaur

The *Six Steps to Effective Management* series comes at a time when the speed and extent of change within health care have rarely been greater, and the challenges facing nurses and everyone working within the health care sector are extensive. The series identifies and discusses those challenges and suggests ways of managing them. It aims to be unique in that it links theory with practice through the application of evidence where available and includes case studies which build on sound and relevant theoretical material.

All nurses are required by the clinical governance agenda to have a grasp of management principles. The *Six Steps to Effective Management* series is both practical enough to appeal to the practitioner and theoretical enough to be useful to those undertaking courses at undergraduate or diploma level. The books are relevant to all nurses.

The series comprises six volumes that are carefully constructed to contain a mix of theoretical and practical approaches, research and case studies, including a variety of perspectives from different sectors of health care. Each volume is relevant, realistic and practical to encourage reflection and critical thinking to prepare readers for flexible and adaptable styles of management.

For more information on this series please contact the Harcourt Health Sciences Health Professions Marketing department on +44 20 7424 4200 (tel).

Contents

Contents

Contents

Contributors

Julia Bradbury FCCA
Finance Manager, Bradford Hospitals Trust, Bradford Royal
Infirmary, Bradford

Angeline Burke BA(Hons) Social Science PGDip Social Research
Methodology
Senior Policy Officer, Association of Community Health
Councils for England and Wales, London

Michael J Cook Ed D (Educational Leadership) MSc(Education
Management) MSc(Quality Management) RGN DipN(Lond) CertEd
Associate Dean, Faculty of Health, St Martin's College,
Lancaster

Ronald W De Witt MA BA(Hons) DipN RCpN RN
Chief Executive, King's College Hospital, London

Brian Edwards CBE FHSM CBIM HonFRCPath D.Univ
Professor of Health Care Development, University of Sheffield,
SCHARR, Sheffield

Con Egan PFA
Chief Executive, Bradford Community Health NHS Trust,
Leeds Road Hospital, Bradford

Helen Fields RGN MEd BEd(Hons) RNT
Head of Education and Registration, NHS Executive,
Headquarters, Department of Health, Leeds

Steve Gosling BA(Hons) DPA(Lond) MSc
Senior Development Manager, NHS Executive, Headquarters,
Department of Health, Leeds

Margaret Goose MA(Cantab) FHSM Hon MFPHM
Chief Executive, The Stroke Association, London

Ros Gray RGN DPSN BN(Hons) PGDip
Clinical Effectiveness Facilitator, Nuffield Hospitals, Education
Centre, Birmingham

M John Hudson MSc CertEd CBiol MIBiol FIBMS MBIM FRSA
Dean, School of Healthcare Studies, University of Leeds, Leeds

Eva M Lambert FCCA
Chief Executive, Pennell Initiative for Women's Health,
Huddersfield

Linda Nazarko MSc BSc(Hons) RN
Director of Nursing, Nightingale Institute, London

Christa M Paxton
Christa M Paxton Associates, London

Richard Romaniak IPFA BSc(Hons)
Finance Manager, Bradford Hospitals NHS Trust, Bradford
Royal Infirmary, Bradford

Rose Stephens RGN DMS MA Health Studies
Chief Nurse Director of Patient Care, Bradford Hospitals NHS
Trust, Bradford

Linda M Terry BA(Hons) PGCE DipM MCIU
Assistant Director, Academic and Business Services,
Department of Health Studies, University of York, York

Carol A Wilby RGN
Business Manager, Education and Regulation, NHS Executive,
Department of Health, Leeds

APPLICATION CONTRIBUTORS

Marion Andrews-Evans RGN BA(Hons) MBA MIMgt
LHG General Manager/Director of Nursing, Gwent Health
Authority, Mamhilad Park, Pontypool

Julia Bradbury FCCA
Finance Manager, Bradford Hospitals Trust, Bradford Royal
Infirmary, Bradford

William J Bryans FCIS FHSM
Specialist Writer on Public Administration, Business and
Finance

Robert Dredge BSc MSc CPFA
Director of Resources, Dudley Health Authority, Dudley, West
Midlands

Marilyn Ekers BA(Hons) AHSM
Senior Policy Manager, NHS Executive (Northern & Yorkshire
Regional Office), Durham

Dame Jill Ellison OBE RGN HV Cert DMS
Nursing Director, Heartlands Hospital, Birmingham

Gayle A Garland RN MSN
Programme Director, Centre for the Development of Nursing
Policy and Practice, University of Leeds, Leeds

Julie Gray RGN DipHSM
Sister, St Luke's Hospital, Bradford Hospitals NHS Trust,
Bradford

Julie Hyde BA(Hons) RGN RCNT RNT CertEd(FE) CERTHSM FRSH
MIHM MIMgt M.ILT
Education, Policy and Management Consultant

Eva M Lambert FCCA
Chief Executive, Pennell Initiative for Women's Health,
Huddersfield

Jo Ouston
Principal, Jo Ouston & Co, London

Contributors

Six Steps to **Effective Management**

Christa M Paxton
Christa M Paxton Associates, London

Gill Poole RGN
Matron, The Wolverhampton Nuffield Hospital,
Wolverhampton

Richard Romaniak IPFA BSc(Hons)
Finance Manager, Bradford Hospitals NHS Trust, Bradford
Royal Infirmary, Bradford

Martin Shreeve BAQEcom DipSW MBA
Programme Director, Better Government for Older People,
Wolverhampton Science Park, Wolverhampton

Rose Stephens RGN DMS MA Health Studies
Chief Nurse Director of Patient Care, Bradford Hospitals NHS
Trust, Bradford

Peter Westhead RMN
Registration and Inspection Officer, Head of Unit, Registration
and Inspection Unit, Leeds Health Authority, Leeds

Carol A Wilby RGN
Business Manager, Education and Regulation, NHS Executive,
Department of Health, Leeds

Sue Williams OBE RSCN RGN DipN(Lond) BEd(Hons)
Nurse Adviser, Greater Glasgow Health Board, Dalian House,
Glasgow

Foreword

The NHS is a huge, complex organisation. It employs one in twenty of all working people in the UK and its turnover – currently £44 billion per annum – exceeds British Airways, British Telecom and Marks & Spencer added together. Everyone in the UK depends on the NHS at some point in their life.

To be successful, the NHS requires highly trained and skilled staff working in teams to ensure safe, effective and high quality services. It also requires good management.

Over the past ten years, it has become quite natural for clinicians to take on leadership and management responsibilities in the NHS. Clinical credibility and management acumen are a powerful combination which leads to strategic and operational improvements in the service.

The Six Steps to Effective Management series emphasises the benefits for staff and patients of working within a framework of continuous quality improvement and professional development. It promotes partnership working and combines theory with examples of good practice in an accessible way.

2001   Sir Alan Langlands

Preface

This book forms part of a series that addresses issues in health care today. Over recent years many changes have occurred which have required all those working in the health industry to be flexible and innovative in order to meet the ever-changing demands of the service. In order to ensure that all users of health and social services receive the best and most appropriate care, managers and clinicians need to be able to react to changes in central policy and interpret this to meet the specific needs of the local population. To do this, professionals from all disciplines need to be able to integrate the spirit of new initiatives and work in real partnerships with a range of agencies to ensure the delivery of seamless care, based upon the best evidence available.

This book is divided into three themes: policy to set the scene, operational perspectives to deliver the business, and quality as a management agenda. When writing this book, both the authors and the editors faced significant challenges. The idea for the series was conceived towards the end of the period of the internal market model of health care delivery, when managers and professionals alike were encouraged to develop qualities of competitiveness in order that their 'product' may take and hold its place in the market. As the business of health care was to a large extent a new concept for many working in the health industry, the business side of the job was an unfamiliar one. Then, about a third of the way through the preparation of the material for the book, the administration changed with the general election in May 1997.

It soon became apparent that the world of health care management was changing. The rhetoric was to end the internal market, and replace competition with partnerships and joint working. Initially it was assumed that the purchaser/provider relationships would be disbanded fully, but it became apparent that this was not to be, as to revert to a world of uncertain financial

Preface

accountability did not make sense. This, of course, meant that the focus in some of the book material was dated before it had been submitted to the publisher. Even people working right at service grassroots reported that change was so rapid that new policy was being sent down the system before the ink was dry. Then the issue of devolution began to gain momentum and it became apparent that the series needed to reflect the different perspectives in the four UK countries. But as we were writing the book at the same time as policy was being developed, this was a challenge!

This fast-changing world is and will be the reality in health care, and in the world generally. Change does not slow up for the authors and editors to capture a particular focus in the book. So when you read this, be aware of this process and time frame. We believe it important that there is a record of many of the processes which have been the basis for the development of health care today and tomorrow. Thus key context issues have been included, even though they may not be 'leading edge' at the time you are reading the book. As health care in the twenty-first century evolves, it is apparent that many principles of the internal market are remaining in a softened format – the pendulum is settling in the middle.

Each chapter of this book aims to provide robust, up-to-date information to encourage readers to think around their experience and think through the issues in the workplace. It is a book that you may wish to read from cover to cover, but more likely, it is a book to dip in to to enable you to meet your particular need; for example to prepare a business plan, or to find a source of voluntary finance. All chapters have been written by authors who are well known and well respected in their field, and their contribution of both time and belief in the value of a series such as this is appreciated. Chapters are followed by short applications, which, in different formats, aim to help the reader make sense of the main themes and principles contained in the chapter.

The concept of clinical governance is the basis for health care delivery at the beginning of the twenty-first century, and this is evidenced in The NHS Plan. It requires that managers and clinical professionals work together in partnerships to ensure that the public receives fit for purpose, quality care provision making best use of resources. This book should assist readers make their contribution by providing the information required to function within the fast-changing business arena of the health industry.

Julie Hyde
Frances Cooper

Section **One**

THE BROAD CONTEXT OF HEALTH CARE

OVERVIEW

Three factors make it important that those involved with the delivery of health care in the UK are aware of the broader context of health care. First, health care is not delivered in a vacuum – the patients and the staff live in a changing society, and thus these changes will impinge upon the way we view our health care systems. Secondly, health care is a political issue. Elections are fought, and won or lost, on the back of health policy. As this edition goes to press, Tony Blair, the prime minister, has announced a tranche of new policy directives, with promises of more money, more staff and better service. It is no coincidence that this term of government is approaching its end – we are beginning the run up to another general election. The third factor is that, even outwith the political debate on the relationship between Great Britain and mainland Europe, we cannot ignore the fact that the world is a smaller place. As people move about to live and work, inevitably they will come across different systems of health provision, and make comparisons – and those are often the catalyst for change.

Thus the first section in this book addresses the big picture. Ron De Witt in Chapter 1 stresses the business element of health, and addresses how this is managed in mainland Europe and beyond. Gayle Garland's application focuses on the core element of business – how health care is funded. She has worked in the USA and has experienced the impact of different funding modules in her own work.

Closer to home, Chapter 2 gives a commentary on current policy drivers, and how the organisational structures have developed to support these. The issue of devolution is introduced here, and followed through in the applications, via snapshots of different development in Scotland, Northern Ireland and Wales. As this book has been in preparation, policy has been evolving, and thus there will be things you find that are now different. This is inevitable because of the run-in time in preparing and printing books, and it does emphasise the point that to keep right up to date with current policy the journals and the government publications are the most appropriate route. Books can give you the background and the theory which support fundamental themes, but will not contain today's news. You may like to look at government publications from your own country, as there are differences in structures and terminology in the four UK countries.

One theme that is common to all is the belief that a quality service is at the heart of health care in the UK, both in the NHS and in the independent sector. Brian Edwards' Chapter 3 gives a focused overview of quality as interpreted within the framework of clinical governance. To demonstrate how policy might be formed at a strategic level via a review of services, then crafted into a document capturing a range of stakeholders' interests which aims to shape the delivery of services, Peter Westhead gives a summary of an important report.

The broad context of health care

Chapter **One**

Health care as a business

Ron De Witt

OVERVIEW

This chapter aims to make two points: (1) that health care, in common with most other organisations or professions, is a business in that it is working within a finite budget (of whatever size) and (2) that the boundaries of health care as we know it in the UK are getting pushed back all the time. Free movement and the right to work within the European Community will have significant effects upon and implications for many people, including of course those working with health. Ron De Witt takes us through the health arrangements of a number of European countries, and points out some comparisons of funding. He then gives a thumbnail sketch of the key characteristics which defined and shaped the internal market, and how these have informed and shaped 'the third way' in the new NHS.

Throughout the 1980s and 1990s in the United Kingdom successive governments have sought to introduce a more business-like approach to many of the organisations and services under direct government control. Such an approach was justified on the grounds that the failure (as perceived by the government) of state-owned and state-managed services was a result of their total immunity to market forces.

Having decided upon a business-orientated approach to address these various organisational shortcomings, the UK government chose to sell off particular industries. They privatised the nationalised industries of gas, electricity, oil, water, coal mining, along with the telecommunications and rail services, with the overall aim of removing the dependence of these sectors on central government financial support.

Where the government decided that the privatisation pathway was not an option which would be supported at the ballot box by the electorate, they followed an entirely different course of action. This was the case for the National Health Service (NHS) and the British Broadcasting Corporation (BBC), with the government choosing to introduce a more business-like approach into the daily activities of these organisations by legislative means, rather than wholesale privatisation. What followed was a period of great change for these services as they strived to meet government targets for performance.

The intention of this chapter is to explore the dynamic between health care and a business-based management approach, utilising examples from around the world where appropriate to develop understanding of why such changes came about. The chapter will also consider the impact of such changes and close with a summary of the present government's intention to bring to an end the 'internal market' for health in the NHS.

BUSINESS AND HEALTH CARE – UNLIKELY BED FELLOWS?

If one were able to rerun history without the political dimension which so influenced health care in the 1990s in the UK, it is highly likely that a number of 'business concepts' would have found their way into the world of health care. The reasons for this are varied but are mainly due to the rapidly changing business environment within which world economies are operating.

Today, the business culture pervades all walks of life. Charles Handy (1994) in his book *The Empty Raincoat* describes how the business ethos has now invaded all aspects of our everyday life:

> Everything is now thought of as a business of a sort. We are all 'in business' these days, be we doctor or priest, professor or charity-worker. *Every* organisation is, in practice, a business because it is judged by its effectiveness in turning inputs into outputs for its customers or clients, and is judged in competition against its peers. The only difference is that 'social businesses' do not distribute their surpluses. (p. 129)

For organisations within Britain such as schools, hospitals and medical practices this means that performance is judged by their effective use of resources and how successful they are in competing for customers.

Commercial businesses vary in size and complexity, they possess a range of common characteristics. These include a predefined purpose, a need to generate profits, provide returns to shareholders, utilise various forms of organisational structure, employ managers, develop business plans and corporate contracts to convey their purpose and clarify to whom they belong. Such characteristics appear to contrast sharply with NHS health care organisations which are social and not economic in nature, driven by the needs of the public's health. However, whilst the principal focus of such commercial organisations is economic return, we would be wrong to dismiss the relevance of all capitalist business approaches purely on the basis that the NHS is not for profit.

Many people, when they talk about health and business in Britain, articulate the case as to why the two are not compatible. They argue that the vast majority of citizens believe that ill health is not something that can be placed second to profit. However, we believe that whilst it is correct to place humanitarian need before profit, to disregard all aspects of business management from the provision of health care is both wrong and impossible to achieve.

The reasoning behind this belief can be attributed to the fact that health care cannot be practised in a vacuum, away from the many factors that impact upon the social and economic standing of a country. Such factors have driven health care reforms in many countries across the world and the UK is no different. Secondly, as Charles Handy described in *The Empty Raincoat* (Handy 1994), the business ethic is already present in all walks of life and health care is no different from any other

Health care as a business

service industry. What is required, however, is a deeper under-standing of the business ethic to appreciate both the relationship and the untapped potential that lies within the health care and business dynamic.

Many people dismiss too readily the suitability of business methods from the world of health care without fully under-standing the many different forms of business that exist, many of which have something to contribute. Albert Michel (1993) in his book *Capitalism against Capitalism* describes three forms of capitalism: Anglo-Saxon or American capitalism, the Continental European version of capitalism and Asian capital-ism, also called 'Confucian' capitalism. Much can be learnt from the Asian variant which has at its heart the 'Chinese contract', a contract that exists between six different stakeholders: financiers, employees, suppliers, customers, environment and society. This hexagon-type contract offers the opportunity to change the priorities of a business to match them with the needs of others. It contrasts sharply with the Anglo-Saxon variant of capitalism, which is focused only upon economic return.

It is essential to acknowledge the various forms of business and the differing philosophies behind them if the potential contribution business may make to health is not to be dis-regarded due to dogma. Acknowledgement of these differing forms of business is also useful in understanding why so many countries across the world have introduced business concepts into their health care provision. Clearly, a business philosophy based on the 'Confucian' philosophy has room to acknowledge the social aspects of health care. This is a topic to which we will return later in this chapter, when consideration is given to the latest health care reforms to be introduced into the NHS.

Further evidence to support the viewpoint of Charles Handy that the business ethic has already pervaded all aspects of everyday life is provided by Robbins (1990), who defines 'an organisation' in terms of four components:

1. *Social entity*   This describes the unit within which people interact in a premeditated way to ensure that critical tasks are completed. As a consequence the need to coordinate the interactions of people arises.
2. *Identifiable boundaries*   Whilst the boundary may change over time, it always distinguishes members from non-members. It tends to be achieved by a contract between members and their organisation, which generally takes the form of an employment agreement and pay. However, in

The broad context of health care

some organisations, such as voluntary and social organisations, the return for individuals may well be prestige, social interaction or the satisfaction of helping others. Every organisation has a boundary that differentiates who is and who is not part of that organisation.

3. *Continuing bond*   This describes the continuing relationship between organisation and individual and the regularity of that bond.

4. *Goals*   All organisations 'exist to do something'. These are termed goals and can be achieved either individually or more effectively as a collective. To achieve these ends members are required to support the mission of the organisation.

These characteristics are common to all organisations and they pervade all aspects of our daily lives. They are the dominant forms of interaction occurring throughout our society in, for example, manufacturing industry, hospitals, schools and retailing. All of these organisations have developed their philosophical base throughout the twentieth century and it should be no surprise that business ideas, philosophies and structures have passed from one sector to another, including health care.

A BRIEF EUROPEAN PERSPECTIVE

Further evidence for the infiltration of business ethics into the world of health care can be seen throughout the European health care system. The different ways in which countries plan and organise their health services appear to vary widely across Europe. However, in the present economic and political climate, planners of health services are being compelled to look closely at ways and means of providing services cheaply without loss of quality. Tremblay (1994) states that 'Although state financial systems and compulsory insurance systems within different member countries looked very different only a few years ago, there are currently several identifiable tendencies within these various systems which are blurring the differences between them.'

Before we consider the impact of the business ethic on the NHS, we will briefly consider the impact within Europe on issues of health care planning and delivery. This will enable us to identify some of the common links between different

Health care as a business

7

European health care systems and broaden our understanding of why similar changes manifested themselves within the health care reforms in the UK during the 1990s.

European countries appear to share similar objectives in their health care policies. Drawing on the work of Barr (1990) these include:

- equal access by patients
- freedom of choice in selecting a doctor or hospital
- cost control at the macro-economic and micro-economic levels
- competition through freedom in determining quality and prices.

However, no health care systems can provide all four of these important design features or values at the same time, and therefore decisions must be made about which features are to be prioritised within a country. This consideration is unique to each country and explains how different countries have evolved different health care systems that are appropriate to their individual histories and important social values.

In general, all European health systems share the same concern with regard to accessibility and equity, but take very different views on financing and the instruments of service delivery. This can be observed in, for example, the approaches to health care in The Netherlands, Sweden, Spain and Portugal.

The Netherlands

The Netherlands introduced a system of health care in the 1990s which is based upon regulated competition between providers, with a strong emphasis upon efficiency and equity. To understand the reasons behind this change in the Dutch health care system it is necessary to understand some of the major milestones in its evolution. Until 1974 the Dutch health care system had a great deal of autonomy; costs were low in terms of gross domestic product (GDP) and growth in the economy was sufficient to meet the increased needs of the population. As a result, government involvement was minimal. However, between 1974 and 1987 the government needed to control state expenditure and therefore introduced policies which set out to restrict the autonomy of the health care system in an attempt to contain costs. At this time, as in Britain, centralised bureaucratic measures were introduced in an attempt to regulate prices and manage service capacity. The result was unsatisfactory. Whilst cost containment was achieved by pursuing cost reduction strategies, these resulted in a demoralised workforce. In practice, the health care system in Holland in the early 1980s was complex, fragmented and costly.

Since 1987, following the publication of the Dekker Committee Report (1987), the Dutch health care system has seen a period of evolution based upon cost effectiveness and efficiency, whilst maintaining the social care values of Dutch society. Throughout this period, health care in Holland has continued to be provided by independent private hospitals, financed mainly through insurance systems. Access to secondary care is through a general practitioner system, although some consumers have the power to purchase directly.

Following the international trend towards less state and more market regulation, the Dutch government introduced an 8-year programme of health care change. The values upon which the changes were formulated are the right of access to health care irrespective of income, combined with a focus on cost effectiveness and efficiency. The changes are summarised in Box 1.1.

The Dutch have pursued a strong line in quality and consumer power, along with further opportunities to achieve efficiency, by allowing competition between providers and purchasers within a regulated health care market. Changes in the funding methodology have resulted in a much more business-like management approach. Providers have obtained more room for self-governance and consequently they behave much more like for-profit organisations. This has required improvements in business management, use of marketing strategies, a

Health care as a business

Box 1.1   Changes in the Dutch health care system in the 1990s

- Service providers lost the right to automatic entitlement to funding. Insurers can now differentiate between providers on the basis of cost and quality.
- Consumers were given greater powers of choice within the new system and clear procedures for the treatment of complaints.
- Steps were taken to strengthen and eliminate perverse incentives in the insurance-based funding scheme for health care.
- Limited deregulation of the health care market was introduced, characterised by lower levels of central government intervention in the provision of health care.

greater focus on efficiency and a keenness to reduce costs; all of which are typical features of the business world.

Sweden

Sweden spends approximately 9% of its GDP on health care. This places it well above the average country in terms of investment. The source of these funds is the public purse and the government contributes some 90% of the health costs. Whilst there is an element of private provision in the Swedish system, nearly all hospitals are owned by the local authorities. This public configuration of provision reflects the high level of priority attached to health care by the Swedish people.

However, despite this high level of investment and priority, problems remain within the Swedish health system. Waiting lists exist for particular treatments, a strong emphasis on hospital-based care is evident and services are not organised to meet consumer requirements. These problems, along with evidence of service inefficiencies, have prompted a reappraisal of service investment patterns along with a review of service costs to seek out inefficiencies.

Since 1991 a number of changes in health care provision have been introduced. These changes have built upon service features that were considered to be non-negotiable:

● a commitment to equity,
● continuation of a tax-based system for funding, and
● continuation of national planning.

One of the main features of the changes to the Swedish system has been the bringing together of health financing and social insurance, focusing upon the emphasis on patient choice, use of competition to stimulate efficiency and the need for effective management to safeguard care and quality of service.

The emergence of a competition-based health care system in a country which has been the model of social democracy is further evidence of not only the application of business ethics within health care systems, but also its apparent suitability for even the most social democratic of societies.

Spain

Spain is currently undergoing a process of political decentralisation. It is intended that this process will introduce improved access to health care, including universality of coverage across the regional systems that are emerging. There is likely to be some restriction on patient choice however.

The compulsory health system is funded by a mix of general taxation and social insurance contributions. This funding is at present managed by the seven autonomous regions of Spain which have health care responsibilities, out of the total of 17 health regions which will take on this role. There is considerable private sector involvement, with 60% of hospitals, for example, being private, for profit. These hospitals receive their funding through contracts with both private insurers and the public sector payers. There is, however, considerable interest in solving the same problems as other countries in terms of searching for better value for money, seeking improvements in clinical efficiency and effectiveness.

The reforms in Spain place the responsibility for regulation and planning of the health system with central government, whilst the regions have responsibility for administering services within each of their geographical areas. The reforms parallel what is happening in other countries but reflect the importance of separating overall responsibilities characteristic of federal states. Particular emphasis has been placed on promoting cost consciousness through greater managerial responsibility. Health commissioning or purchasing will continue to be separate, but there will be efforts to define a common core service requirement.

Clear evidence exists to support the premise that Spain is utilising business management techniques to address the shortcomings of their health system.

Portugal

Since 1975, when private and voluntary hospitals were nationalised, Portugal has operated a national health service designed to integrate the various health resources into a coherent whole. The political system of Portugal puts significant power in the hands of the central state, but the regions have the main responsibility for ensuring that services available are fully integrated to the benefit of the patient.

General taxation funds the system, but there is still some independent activity which must be compatible with national objectives. The Portuguese national health service has evolved since 1975 to a system which, originally designed to be free, now involves co-payment based on the ability to pay or on income.

Health care as a business

Portugal is also keen to ensure increased competition between the public and private sectors to improve efficiency and to ensure that consumers have freedom of choice. Funding of hospitals, for example, has moved from global budgets, to funding based on the analysis of costs of treatments for different diagnosis-related groups. Progressive contracting out of services from the largely state-owned hospitals to the few remaining private hospitals and service providers is a newer initiative intended to encourage the desired competition.

Features of the European-wide health care system

The four models of health care described briefly above have been chosen to illustrate some of the differing approaches to health care provision within Europe today. Some countries have rejected national health systems because their own approaches have evolved from an insurance-orientated structure which has fitted with the particular values of that country. These countries leave the role of government to set the rules of the health service through insurance funds, which in some countries are locally controlled, working with doctors and hospitals to meet the needs of the patients.

However, regardless of which system of health care financing is used there is, as identified by Tremblay (1994), common ground upon which all European health care is founded. The principles are summarised in Box 1.2.

> **Box 1.2** Principles of health care common to all European countries
>
> - A system based on a set of social values including equity, access for all and income protection against health costs based on the ability to pay.
> - A desire to see health care expenditure consume an appropriate share of a nation's wealth (gross domestic profit).
> - Intention to maximise improvements in health to the satisfaction of the public given the resources available for health care.
> - Freedom of choice for consumers.
> - The involvement of third party coverage.
> - Reliance upon compulsory insurance or taxes to fund health services.

In the European examples cited, each was facing problems with regard to health care provision. These countries are not unique in this respect; at present throughout Europe all countries are facing similar problems. However, what would appear to be unique is that in responding to these challenges the various approaches they are adopting all have at their core strong business principles. This approach is characterised by the use of regulated market reform to deliver improvements in the effectiveness and efficiency of their health care systems.

In many parts of Europe the issue of bringing together business and health care is clearly not the same issue it is in the UK. In many European countries the national culture and values readily accept the necessity of a focused business management approach. This is true today even in Sweden for example, where the national culture may have prevented such developments a few years ago. However this is not the case in the UK.

The greatest external influence on any future UK health system is likely to originate from within Europe and not from North America, and membership of the European Union is bound to have a significant impact on the British health care system. The main effects of the European Union to date have been felt in relation to trade and industry. Its effect on the social perspective has been limited to workers' rights and their position within organisations. However, all of this changed with the Maastricht Treaty in 1991, which gave the Union the right to engage in foreign affairs, defence and social policy. The original decision of the UK government at that time to reject the Social Chapter has been overturned by the present government, who intend to implement in full the detail contained within the Treaty and the Social Chapter during the legislative programme.

The initial impact of the Maastricht Treaty on issues of health will be felt in terms of future health legislation within the European Community. We will return to this issue of Europe in the final section of this chapter.

UK HEALTH CARE REFORM IN THE 1990s

The UK health system, like its European equivalents, has undergone a series of changes during the 1990s. However, these changes must be seen in the context of the deep affection that the people of Britain have for the NHS. For many people, the creation of the NHS was the greatest piece of social legislation in the 20th century, and was even more remarkable considering it was undertaken at a time when other countries were concentrating on priorities of economic regeneration (following World War II) rather than social progress. Equally, the NHS is a great success story. It is a low cost service compared to other western health care systems. For example, in The Netherlands expenditure on health service accounted for 8.5% of GDP, in Ireland, 5.5% of GDP, whereas in Britain it was just 4.0% of GDP (Hurst 1992) and yet most indicators of health in the UK are at least as good as in many other western nations spending far more than the British government (1999 figures suggest 6.9% of GDP is spent on health in the UK (Yuen, 2000)). This success breeds an unwillingness to look carefully at how further improvements can be made and a refusal to question 'sacred cows'. Health care is one of the world's largest industries and the NHS is the largest within that industry. Even against the background of recession it is a growth industry. Challenges must be met, change must occur to meet the challenges of today's world, but it must be remembered that the NHS is a 'sacred cow' which is accountable to the nation.

If the NHS was such a successful organisation why then did the government of Margaret Thatcher seek to introduce a series of fundamental changes during the early 1990s? The answer to this lies partly with the political philosophy of the Conservative Party, characterised by its focus upon wholesale privatisation of state-run service industries, a commitment to reduce reliance upon central government support and the aim of creating consumer-sensitive organisations, focused on outcomes. The remainder of the answer as to why change was required lies within the NHS itself. Although, as has been said, it was and still is very successful relative to health care systems in other countries, it also faced the same problems as other countries, the solutions to which required a period of change.

The need for change

Various drivers for change faced by the NHS in the late 1980s and early 1990s can be identified.

Cost control

Health care costs became and remain a dominant theme in most western countries. Purchasers are under real pressure to demand of providers continued improvements in efficiency, so that money can be released for service developments. Nevertheless, escalating funding demands are made as a result of an ageing population, new diagnostic and therapeutic technologies, as well as demands for better conditions for staff.

Value for money

It has long been recognised that more money is not necessarily the solution to the problems of the NHS. Excessive use of institutional services instead of the development of community-based alternatives, overprescribing of drugs, better health education are just a few examples of more effective but cheaper options (Audit Commission Report 1993, p. 6). Often, additional funding only delays the development of appropriate professional mechanisms and of planning structure and process to enable change.

Lack of professional accountability

Health professionals, particularly doctors, have traditionally accepted accountability for the quality of outcomes of clinical care. However, prior to the reforms they denied accountability for collective decision making for cost outcomes, balance of care and/or care of the wider community. Each doctor tended to function as an individual in competing for services and patients; this ultimately had a negative impact on the health care system.

Imbalances of care

Medical specialisation is well defined in most developed countries and has become more so in the last decade as a result of advanced technology and knowledge. As specialties and services changed, some were seen to slip behind others and become disadvantaged. Disquiet at this state of affairs was voiced by the general public and consumer groups such as MIND and Age Concern.

Health care as a business

15

Despite an ageing population, the high profile and technology-dependent services tend to consume vast amounts of resources. Equally, the acute hospital sector is seen to be cash-rich at the expense of the primary and community care sector.

These drivers for change were not unique to the NHS alone; as stated earlier, other countries in Europe were facing similar problems. Neither were these problems entirely unique to the period. For much of its history, the NHS has appeared to be in a permanent state of crisis which was best summarised by Enoch Powell in 1976, when he said in Parliament:

> One of the most striking features of the NHS is the continual deafening chorus of complaints which rises day and night from every part of it, a chorus only interrupted when someone suggests a different system. The universal Exchequer financing of the service endows everyone providing as well as using it with a vested interest in denigrating it.

The chorus of complaint to which Powell refers has continued unabated despite significant increases in expenditure, staff employed and patients treated. During the 1980s the government of the day focused its attention on the management arrangements of the NHS. This resulted in the 1983 management inquiry led by Sir Roy Griffiths (1983). At the time of the inquiry many people believed that 'management', with its connotations of setting health service activities into an economic context, had no real place in the health service and certainly the professions ought not to be involved. Since the early days of the NHS, the role of government was seen to be the provider of funding and it was felt that the health professionals should be free within the constraints of that funding to set their own priorities largely based on clinical decisions.

Griffiths concluded that the machinery of translating policy into action and generally of effecting change was extremely limited. Recommendations were made with regard to establishing a system of management within the NHS that would offer leadership and the means to monitor, review and manage NHS performance. However, the report faced a 'catch-22' situation in that it was asking for a full management process to be introduced when there was little management to introduce it.

Implementation of the recommendations also proved to be difficult because of the funding crisis facing the NHS in the mid-1980s and the high levels of professional resistance to the report. Indeed the medical profession viewed the report, with its emphasis on management, as a distraction from the real problem of the NHS, lack of funding. The funding problems reached their height in 1987 when the Royal Colleges warned the government that the NHS was in terminal decline. The prime minister's response was to establish her own review. Whilst this review started with a focus upon NHS funding, it was made clear that certain features of the service were seen to be non-negotiable. These included the provision of services free at the point of delivery and the financing of the service through general taxation.

The prime minister's review set the agenda for health from 1989 onwards, with many of its recommendations being encapsulated within the legislative programme of the 1990s. The main elements of the reforms are listed in Box 1.3.

Following these reforms there were a series of changes in the central management structure of the NHS designed to enable it to fulfil its strategic management role. In 1994 a streamlining of central management occurred. This created a clear identity for the NHS Management Executive, within the Department of Health as the headquarters of the NHS. This identity has been strengthened by the abolition of the 14 statutory Regional Health Authorities and reorganising the Executive to include eight regional offices. At more local levels, a greater identity for purchasing and a mechanism for control of resources has led to the merging of DHAs and FHSAs to create stronger local purchasers.

Box 1.3   Main elements of the NHS reforms of the 1990s

- The establishment of NHS Trusts.
- The introduction of GP fundholders. These GPs had the funds to purchase certain hospital services and treatments for their patients.
- The development of the purchasing function. District Health Authorities (DHA) were charged with assessing the health needs of their local population and purchasing the services most appropriate to those needs from a range of service providers.
- The encouragement of closer working relationships between DHAs and Family Health Service Authorities (FHSA) to ensure a better balance between hospital and community health services and primary care services.

Health care as a business

Impact of the reforms

Turning now to consider the impact of the reforms on the NHS during the period 1990–1997, a number of issues can be identified.

Lack of coordination

Despite the NHS reforms there continued to be a wide range of agencies involved in patient service provision. It could be said that the numbers of provider organisations have increased as a consequence of the reforms. For example, GP fundholders (GP fundholding institutions) and local councils (under the Care in the Community Act, 1994) became provider organisations.

The main impact of this fragmentation is the obstacle it places in the way of a holistic view of patient services being undertaken. The fragmentation confines chunks of patient services to managerial institutions and prevents the establishment of integrated care models. In practice, services cannot be planned without taking account of both the physical boundaries and the self-interest of both hospitals and social communities.

Change and the rate of change

Organisations and institutions in health and social systems, especially non-profit entities, are often highly resistant to change. Klein (1976) refers to this as 'organisational sclerosis'. In health, this problem is related to historical precedents, parochialism, lack of change management skills and conflict between health professionals and managers. It is further compromised by funding and management of health services along hierarchical institutionalised lines, a problem that has been increased by the NHS reforms and the creation of, for example, Acute Trusts, Community Trusts and Ambulance Trusts. Not only were problems encountered in relation to establishing these organisations, but the self-preservation instincts of these organisations have presented further difficulties in relation to service change. In practice, this means that where the consensus view is that services could be improved by merging particular organisations or by moving service provision from one organisation to another, progress in many cases is slow. This lack of progress leads to frustration and, in some instances, poor decisions as a process of horse trading is initiated to satisfy the expectations and needs of the organisations and staff concerned.

In the early days of the reforms much was made of impact that the speed of change and lack of relevant information was likely to have on the success of the changes to be made. This was especially true for GP fundholding, with the Royal Colleges and the British Medical Association calling for a period of piloting to test the proposals before national roll out. This call was rejected by the government, much to the annoyance of the professional bodies concerned. It is probably worth comparing at this stage the very different approaches to change adopted by our European partners. In Holland, the 1990 coalition government, building upon the 1987 Dekker Report, sought to adopt an evolutionary and not revolutionary approach to the issue of health care reform. An 8-year time frame was developed to enable managed change to occur. In Sweden, once the need to change was accepted, the crossroads project did not set out to produce specific recommendations for change, but to detail scenarios/options for the future. These in turn have been picked up by two government commissions who were charged with managing the debate and seeking to establish the best way forward based upon the values of Swedish society.

Reasons behind the rapid rate of change in Britain are probably related to political imperatives (the next general election was due in 1992) and the particular personalities involved in the government of the day. Either way, the speed of change did no real favours to the NHS in terms of building a consensus behind the merits of the reforms.

Lack of community involvement

The lack of community involvement in the planning of services, self-help and personal care initiatives contributes to the difficulties the general public has in understanding what the NHS does offer and why change is necessary. It could be said that the reforms have distanced the community even further from the policy makers. However, if one is to accept that GP fundholding and health purchasers represent 'patients', then there is more leverage on providers, with the potential to influence change through contracts.

The market

In the early days of reform, much was made of the 'internal market' and the need to encourage competitiveness, efficiency and effectiveness. The intention was to stimulate improvements in the performance of the NHS overall. However, the main outcome was to set NHS Trust against NHS Trust in many parts of the country. This resulted in the perpetuation of self-interest and many NHS Trusts initiated service developments to gain a greater share of the market resource, without any acknowledgement of the wider community needs and the existing services at other Trusts. The competitive theme extended even to the sharing of workforce data, with each NHS Trust refusing to disclose information to another, on the basis that this might provide a neighbouring NHS Trust with a competitive advantage. Such decisions severely restricted the capability of the NHS to function as a national service and led to calls for the internal market to be abolished.

GP fundholding

One of the most common criticisms of the reforms concerned the formation of a two-tier system which resulted from the GP fundholding scheme. Under this scheme general practitioners who opted for fundholding status were able to purchase patient services directly from NHS Trusts. The intention was to enable the purchaser, in this case the GP, to deal directly with the service provider, thereby achieving service efficiencies, improvements in the quality of service and speedier access to patient services. The results were mixed, with individual GPs realising that even under the terms of the fundholding scheme they had little leverage in terms of realising service changes. They did, however, manage to gain the attention of service providers as a consequence of the sums of money they had in their practice budgets, which enabled their patients to gain access to services at times when patients of non-fundholding GPs could not.

Community nursing

The reforms also created a lack of coordination between the various professional staff who deliver the public health agenda in the community setting. As an example, health visitors, school nurses and occupational health therapists all operated independently of each other and at times even in separate parts of the same organisations without any reference to each other's function and contribution.

Contracting process

A further feature of the reforms of the 1990s was the focus on service contracts. Frequently, this has resulted in a line by line analysis of services as described under the terms of the contract. Such an approach has prevented an holistic approach to service delivery being taken in many instances.

This process has also excluded key individuals from particular discussions. The majority of managers and other health professionals are excluded from the medically dominated debate which shapes the public health agenda. They therefore faced great difficulties in knowing how much emphasis to place on different segments of the policy. Equally, few clinicians saw the detail of what was negotiated between the purchaser and provider. This disconnection also resulted in the failure to connect the work patterns of the individual health workers with the public health agenda, which was set by the Health Authorities.

Examples such as these tested the patience of the British public. Many held the view that competitiveness, secrecy and market share were all attributes of the world of business and had no place in the NHS. However, it would be wrong to suggest that the reforms did not deliver some positive features which have enabled the service to move on.

Allocation of resources

As the internal market became established and the public became increasingly aware of the many issues facing the NHS in the 1990s, the issue of resource allocation came increasingly to the fore. Certainly the market economy of health raised the public profile of decisions about the funding of specific specialties and treatments. The impact of this was felt in two ways; first, the fact that decisions were being openly discussed in the public arena generated a greater sense of openness and enabled such decisions to be scrutinised. Second, because these decisions were having to be defended in the public arena, this introduced the concept of 'clinical effectiveness' to the public.

GP fundholding

In the early days of fundholding, those practices who made up the first and second wave practices were seen to be the

Health care as a business

innovators. The advantages offered under the scheme in terms of the perceived shift in power from the hospital consultant to the general practitioner and the opportunity to manage one's own budget certainly attracted those practices who were likely to lead rather than be led. Central guidance offered the opportunity to use savings in one of four ways:

1. Paying for additional staff or hospital services
2. Improving practice premises
3. Improving facilities for patients
4. Providing additional medical equipment.

Savings generated as a consequence of fundholding, and their subsequent use by practices, certainly drew a great many critical comments. This was even harder to defend at the time when other parts of the NHS appeared to be under-resourced. However, placing those arguments to one side, the fact that savings were achievable did demonstrate that placing the responsibility for budgetary expenditure at the primary care level did have a sobering impact on a number of practitioners in terms of their referral patterns.

Fundholding also enabled patient choice to be reaffirmed within the NHS. This was certainly true for those practices which were served by a number of hospitals. Under the terms of the scheme they could offer their patients real choice in terms of the hospital they attended.

Further advantages of the fundholding scheme include the ability of some practices to effect real change in the service arrangements of the hospitals with which they contracted. Examples where changes were effected included the prompt arrival of a satisfactory discharge letter following a hospital episode. Changes such as these often resulted from the discussions held between consultants and general practitioners, a meeting which had occurred in some instances for the very first time and only as a result of fundholding status. Other changes included open access arrangements for some services, such as physiotherapy, and the provision of consultant-led outpatient clinics within health centres.

Outcomes

Overall, it can be seen that the reforms resulted in a variety of outcomes for the NHS. Some aspects of the business-orientated approach were clearly inappropriate to the NHS (e.g. protectionism), whilst others (e.g. improved efficiency in primary care with the generation of practice savings) were to be welcomed. However, since the mid-1990s NHS Trusts and GP fundholders have seen the original freedoms they were given gradually decline, resulting in minimal change and a limiting effect on some of the potentially more radical aspects of the reforms. As a consequence, Trusts have found it increasingly difficult to respond to rapidly developing new situations, with purchasers increasingly demanding service changes over shorter timescales.

Equally, the more competitive elements of the reforms have taken a back seat in recent years, with competitors tending to voluntarily agree (by negotiation) on acceptable levels of market share and acceptable norms of behaviour. This has been characterised in the large cities by the defining of 'strategic alliances' between NHS Trusts.

Throughout the period of the reforms, the focus remained upon waiting lists as a proxy for NHS performance. A number of successes was achieved in reducing the maximum length of stay for inpatient treatment to 18 months, and in recent years considerable effort has been expended to reduce this further to 12 months. However, this position has been difficult to maintain and many opposition MPs during the national election campaign of 1997 used this slippage to highlight the current difficulties of the NHS, attributable in their view to underfunding.

Red tape was also one of the NHS election themes for 1997. Ever since the start of the reforms the creation of an 'internal market in health' was seen by some to be a bureaucrat's dream. The cost of running the NHS 'internal market' was, for many stakeholders, indefensible at a time when decisions were being taken not to purchase particular treatments and many Trusts were running large debts. The costs of the market were attributable to the transaction costs of the various patient episodes and the additional management input required to enable the system to function.

It was no surprise, therefore, that the change in government in May 1997 was accompanied by a series of changes for the NHS. The final section of this chapter will deal briefly with these changes and the potential influence of Europe.

THE NEW NHS

The Labour government's White Paper 'The New NHS: Modern, Dependable', was published in December 1997 (Department of Health 1997). It describes the government's intention to abolish the internal market for health, and to replace it with an integrated care approach. The abolition of the market aims to save £1 billion of red tape, which can then be reinvested in patient services. New hospitals are to be built, and breast cancer and children's services to receive additional money. Emphasis is placed upon improving standards year on year, delivering high quality to all.

So what of business and health care? Will we no longer see business methods applied in the NHS? Early indications are that business methods will still be part of this new NHS, as the White Paper states that the service in the future will be based upon partnership and driven by performance. This new approach to health care is described as the 'third way'. Interestingly, the government, whilst abolishing the internal market aspect of the previous government's reforms, will retain what has worked. Overall this means that the separation between the planning and provision of care will remain. However GP fundholding is to be abolished and all GPs are to be grouped within locally determined Primary Care Groups. In delivering these changes, six important principles guide the process (Box 1.4).

This new approach to health care is a mix of the pre-reform and reform period. The approach accommodates particular aspects of a more business-like approach as a means of improving NHS performance in terms of efficiency and quality. However, this business ethic is not the Anglo-Saxon business variation, with its strong focus upon economic return, as detailed in the first section of this chapter. Such an approach, which was closely associated with the NHS reforms of the early 1990s, has been rejected. The new business approach values the social aspects of business and is more akin to the Chinese form of business, again described in the first section of this chapter.

Box 1.4 Six overriding aims guiding reform of the NHS under Labour

1. To renew the NHS as a genuinely **national** system.
2. To make the delivery of health care against these new national standards a matter of **local** responsibility.
3. To get the NHS to work in **partnership**.
4. To improve **efficiency** so that every pound in the NHS is spent to maximise the care for patients.
5. To shift the focus onto quality of care so that **excellence** is guaranteed to all patients.
6. To rebuild **public confidence** in the NHS.

The new NHS will still be required to balance its books and difficult choices remain in terms of which patient services and particular treatments will be funded. However, the government intends to ensure that across the country, patients have the right of access to similar services. No longer will inequity be acceptable on the basis of funding or geographical location and balancing the books will not be the only imperative which will guide chief executives. Under the new arrangements all have a legal duty for the quality of services delivered within their Trusts.

This new responsibility places quality of care alongside the need to maintain financial balance, and should enable the NHS to demonstrate how it is possible to integrate business ethics into everyday practice. This business ethic will not have the need to generate profit as its sole goal; 'satisfactory care' will also be a goal of equivalent status.

It is still early days in terms of working through the implications of these latest reforms for the NHS and lessons must be learnt from previous experience of reforms. A commonality of understanding and purpose is required for all players in the new NHS. We cannot just place people in rooms and expect them to get on with the changes to be made. The application of management of change principles, with a clear focus upon unity of purpose and accountability, will prove invaluable in terms of meeting national and local objectives, especially for those who have to accept the responsibility for delivery. This responsibility must extend to the social sector, who have a major contribution to make to the general health of the population in terms of housing, education and social care. Whilst this potential contribution is recognised within the White Paper, delivery on the ground will demand national support and local determination to apply business discipline to this process of change. Business is more than just a focus upon money and profit, it is also about applying business practice to the performance of the organisation, including quality of service and the attainment of shared and agreed objectives within and outwith the organisation.

The NHS is now set on a further period of change which is said to be evolutionary and not revolutionary, within a 10-year time frame. Whether the government is willing to stay with this particular 10-year period for change remains to be seen. Certainly recent experience suggests that the political imperative remains high on the agenda and the speed of change may need to be delivered over much shorter timescales if political goals are to be achieved.

Health care as a business

The influence of the European Community on the new NHS

The outcome of translating strategy into actual practice is difficult to predict accurately within any sector, and is especially so in health. Whilst 'The New NHS: Modern, Dependable' (Department of Health 1997) maps out the objectives for the NHS over the period to 2007, we will find the service increasingly influenced by the European Community. As described earlier, the Maastricht Treaty will extend the influence of the European Community into the area of health legislation. Whilst the responsibility for determining the exact nature of the health provision within member countries remains with each national government, the Commission will form a view on the impact of health systems on the public health. Questions on regional inequalities in health will no doubt be high on the agenda.

Since the Maastricht Treaty, the Commission has examined the issue of health and indeed a report was placed before the European Parliament entitled 'Public Health After Maastricht' in October of 1993. This report recommended the formalisation of the Commission's responsibilities with regard to the issue of health. Recommendations within the report included the preparation of policies in a number of areas, including AIDS, cancer screening and drug dependency. This move is a major step in the coordination of health activities across all member states and indicates the need for the NHS to carefully consider European legislation and its potential impact in the UK.

The influence of the European Community in terms of business ethics further confirms that those persons who see no role for business principles in health care are increasingly likely to be swimming against the tide. This is especially so when we have the direct influence of the Commission to consider and the UK government embracing business, by virtue of 'the third way'.

References

Albert M (1993) Capitalism against capitalism. London: Whurr.

Audit Commission Report (1993) Value for money: development in the NHS. London: HMSO.

Barr N (1990) Economic theory and the welfare state: a survey and reinterpretation. Welfare State Programme, Discussion Paper No. 54. London School of Economics and Political Science

Decker Committee (1987) Willingness to change. Government Committee on Health Structure and Financing. Amsterdam.

The broad context of health care

Department of Health (1997) The new NHS: modern, dependable. London: Department of Health.

Griffiths R (1983) The NHS management inquiry report. HC209. London: HMSO.

Handy C (1994) The empty raincoat: the meaning of business. London: Hutchinson.

Hurst J (1992) The reform of health care systems: a comparative analysis of seven OECD countries. Health Policy Studies No. 2. Paris: OECD.

Klein R E (1976) Political cosmetics are no answer. Health and Social Services Journal, 1804–1805. Volume LXXXVI No. 4511

Robbins S (1990) Organisation theory, structure, design and applications. New York: Prentice-Hall.

Tremblay M (1994) Health policy and Europe discussion. Study Guide for Brussels Conference. University of Birmingham.

Yuen P (2000) Compendium of health statistics, 12th edn. London: Office of Health Economics.

Health care as a business

Application 1:1 *Gayle Garland*

The impact of different health care funding models on nursing practice in the USA

This application describes how finance has influenced particular areas of health care delivery in the USA. The principle is one of resource management, and as you use this book you will see that theme emerging again and again. No longer can health care function with 'an open cheque'. Resource management exists in all areas of life, in all countries. A key theme is about partnership between clinicians and general management. In the UK a number of private hospitals now offer fixed price treatment, and we are seeing relationships develop between some private insurance groups and some private hospitals in an effort to manage the resource.

THE EVOLUTION OF FINANCIAL MODELS IN THE US HEALTH CARE SYSTEM

The US health care system is financed very differently to the NHS. Built around the free market strategy, physicians and hospitals are independent contractors who compete for patients and profits. Private and public health insurance are the major funding sources for health services, with Medicare, the federal government health insurance programme for the elderly and disabled, being the largest insurer in the nation. Prior to 1983, consistent with the free market philosophy, insurance payments to hospitals and physicians were based on a fee-for-service or indemnity model. Each day spent in hospital, each diagnostic procedure, and every treatment, including medications and surgery, was reimbursed to providers based on an agreed fee schedule. The economic incentives to hospitals and physicians in this payment system were to keep the patient in hospital for long periods and to conduct as many tests and treatments as possible. As a result, health care became a highly profitable industry for providers, and the purchasers, predominantly insurance companies, faced huge cost increases. Economists and budget analysts forecasted that the level of growth in insurance costs made the indemnity model unsustainable in the future.

In 1983, the US government passed a law introducing the prospective payment system (PPS) for Medicare, which dramatically changed the financial incentives for providers. Prospective payment means that providers are paid a set fee based on the patient's diagnosis regardless of the length of stay in hospital or the costs sustained in the course of care. Under prospective payment, providers are rewarded for treating patients efficiently, with lower costs, fewer tests and treatments and shorter episodes of care. Hospitals were the first providers to be subjected to prospective payment with the government promising to implement the system for physicians and non-acute care providers within a few years of the hospital implementation. Almost 15 years have passed since the implementation of the prospective payment system in hospitals. To date, physician payment from Medicare remains a fee-for-service model. The unfortunate consequence of this situation is that the two principal providers of acute care, physicians and hospitals, have differing incentives. In order to survive, hospitals are placed in the position of policing physician practices for efficiency and cost, a situation which has introduced an adversarial element in what was once a cohesive approach to patient care.

The latest financial model to evolve has been managed care or capitation financing model. Under this system, insurance companies pay physician groups and hospitals based on a 'per member, per month' formula irrespective of the services provided. For example, an insurance company will contract with a hospital to supply any needed care for its members based on a flat fee per month for each person they represent. If all those people remain well during a particular month, the insurance company still pays the hospital the agreed fee even though no services are provided. If two of the insured members have cardiac surgery in the next month, the insurance company still pays the agreed fee even if the real costs to the hospital far outweigh the contracted reimbursement. The same financial incentives apply for physician groups. It is in the best interest of physician groups to keep the patients well, which reduces the cost and results in profit for the practice. In this model, the incentives for providers are to keep the patients well. Profits are directly related to lowest demand for care, especially hospital care.

THE IMPACT OF FINANCIAL MODELS ON NURSING CARE

Much has changed in the delivery of nursing care as a result of the shift in financial models. Under fee-for-service reimbursement, the majority of medical and nursing care occurred in hospital. Community services were underdeveloped and undervalued. Patients could expect a thorough, unhurried course of treatment. In fact, overtreatment was sometimes an issue, and many believe that excessive diagnostic testing was a common occurrence. Nursing within this model was a comfortable, secure job within a prosperous industry.

Prospective payment changed all that. In order to survive, hospitals were forced to improve the efficiency of care. Patients were in hospital for shorter periods and wards started to empty out. The remaining hospital patients were sicker and required more care. Declining budgets and patient populations required innovative staffing patterns. Many hospitals adopted strict staffing ratios, requiring nurses to go home without pay when the patient census dropped. Redundancies were common despite increasing patient acuity on the wards.

Nurses took on new roles. Discharge planning became an area of specialty nursing practice. With the emphasis on discharging patients home 'sicker and quicker', expert preparation was needed. Discharge coordinators ensured that follow-up appointments were made, transportation arranged, medical equipment delivered to the house, family members were educated, and professional nursing services engaged for continuing care. This role evolved in many institutions to include utilisation review wherein nurses became involved in encouraging best practice by physicians. This in turn evolved to case management by nurses which encompasses financial, social, psychological and physical planning for continuing care after discharge from hospital. The need for domiciliary nursing care grew, as did the intensity of nursing care in nursing homes and other non-acute care settings. Nurses aptly modified practice to include these new venues for acute and continuing care.

The trends begun by the shift to prospective payment were supported and accelerated by the recent move toward managed care. Under a managed care model, hospitals and physicians are rewarded for minimising intervention. Best practice is identified as practice which keeps patients well. Emphasis is placed on management of chronic diseases such as diabetes, on prevention through education, on early diagnosis of conditions such as cancers, and on efficient care of those patients who develop acute illnesses. Nurses have responded to these latest developments by embracing new roles as health educators, patient advocates and case managers.

Funding models in the USA

Chapter **Two**

The NHS today

Julie Hyde with Adrian Booth

This chapter was originally written by Elizabeth Gardner but during the preparation of the book, many radical and complex changes have been introduced, and continue, across all sectors of health care provision in the UK. As a result, this chapter, in common with other chapters in the book, has been revised and revisited on a number of occasions. The editors and the publishers are very grateful to all those friends and colleagues who contributed to this process by responding to requests with speed and good humour. Readers, please be aware of the pace of change, and consult the journals, and relevant government publications, in all four UK countries, for the most up-to-date information.

OVERVIEW

Commentators suggest that the NHS has seen more changes since May 1997 than at any other time since its implementation in 1948. The framework for these changes is outlined in this chapter, which also seeks to point out the differences in the four UK countries. However, at the time of going to press, changes are still taking place in all four countries, and readers should be aware of this. 'Managing the business of health care' is not a fixed process. That is why writing about it can be such a challenge! The pace of change is so fast that no text book can be completely up to date, and you are encouraged to read this chapter in the context of the day/week/month in which you are reading it! Weekly journals are useful to flag up very recent changes, and you might like to make a note of new policy decisions, and keep them tucked into the relevant page of the book. A key example is that of the publication of 'The NHS Plan' for England in July 2000 and for Scotland in December 2000. These important documents outline the government's plans to modernise the NHS in order to provide for the public quality, seamless services.

However, one constant factor which is important to glean from this chapter, is that health care is driven by the political agenda. Devolution is a prime example of this, but other issues can impinge, via politics, on health care. A recent incident likely to be recorded as an influential case is the trial of Harold Shipman, the general practitioner convicted, in February 2000, of mass murder. Because of this, there have been a range of political demands made of the medical profession to prevent such a tragedy happening in the future.

This chapter aims to outline the framework of the new NHS following the publication of the government's White Papers which set out changes to the structure and aims of the NHS (Department of Health 1997, Scottish Office Department of Health 1997, Welsh Office 1998a). The decision to deliver health care via devolved government is addressed, although this is ongoing as this text goes to press. The roles, duties, objectives and constraints of the key stakeholders will be explored.

The new NHS is characterised by partnerships, both between key players within the NHS and between the NHS and outside bodies. The move from a competitive health service (i.e. the internal market) to a more collaborative one described by the new NHS will demand new styles of working.

First it is helpful to consider the wider historical context, and to look at the underpinning principles which have resulted in the changes brought about under the heading 'The New NHS'.

The NHS today

Following the change in administration in May 1997 when a Labour government was elected following a long period of Conservative majority, the overall approach to health and social policy changed. From a rather straightforward view of health (i.e. absence of illness) which had, in reality, prevailed for a number of years, the new government took a wider view of health. Their approach is more inclusive, emphasising that health and social policy go hand in hand, and thus should be delivered within partnerships. They believe that health care should take a broad view of health, including all things that have impact on people's health. An example of this would be housing which traditionally has not been addressed within the NHS. This government has focused more on *public health*, addressing ways in which health can be improved for all by addressing inequalities. To do this of course flags up the need for partnerships between a range of organisations, as 'joined-up' problems need 'joined-up' solutions.

This chapter considers the contribution of each part of the NHS in meeting the principles behind the White Papers for England, Wales and Scotland, and the consultation documents considering health care issues in Northern Ireland. These principles state that the NHS will remain a *national* service, incorporating a high degree of *local responsibility* for delivering *quality care*. *Partnerships*, not just between health organisations, but including also local authorities, the voluntary and private sectors, carers and patients, are seen as essential in order to maximise *efficiency* and *performance* and so rebuild *public confidence*.

The English Green Paper 'Our Healthier Nation: a Contract for Health' (Department of Health 1998) was published in 1998 and following consultation, the White Paper 'Saving Lives: our Healthier Nation' (Department of Health 1999a) emerged. In Scotland and Wales, sister White Papers emerged entitled 'Towards a Healthier Scotland' (Scottish Office Department of Health 1999) and 'Better Health – Better Wales' (Welsh Office 1998b). No equivalent was published in Northern Ireland, but the principles of public health have been embraced by health professionals in the Province.

A number of initiatives has rolled from the public health agenda, all of which are captured in The NHS Plan (Department of Health 2000) for England and The Scottish Plan (Scottish Office Department of Health 2000) for Scotland. An equivalent plan for Wales is expected in early 2001 and discussions are underway in Northern Ireland.

Some examples of these initiatives are Social Exclusion Units (see Application 2.1), New Deal Initiatives, Healthy Living

Box 2.1 Key players in the organisation of the NHS

- The government
- Secretary of state/Department of Health
- NHS Executive/Regional Offices
- Health Authorities and Boards
- NHS Trusts
- Primary Care Groups, Local Health Groups, Local Health Care Cooperatives and Primary Care Trusts

Centres, Sure Start and Single Regeneration Budget, all of which rely upon partnerships and modernisation of the health service to deliver to the public.

Thus it is necessary to draw out the relationships between a number of key players, highlighting the importance of mutual commitment if the NHS is to be run effectively (see Box 2.1).

THE GOVERNMENT

Setting the budget

The NHS is funded through general taxation. The initial decision as to how much public expenditure is to be devoted to the NHS is determined by the government and announced by the Chancellor of the Exchequer in a statement to Parliament. In previous years the announcement has followed an annual, 'behind-closed-doors' bidding round by the secretaries of state in each of the major government departments. However, in June 1998 the Chancellor of the Exchequer announced that departments will be given 3-year spending totals.

Separate announcements are made which detail the breakdown of expenditure within the Scottish, Welsh and Northern Ireland Offices. Ultimate responsibility for the resourcing of health care rests with decisions made in the Treasury, based on the competing priorities of each department.

The establishment of the Scottish Parliament and Assemblies for Wales and Northern Ireland have led to decisions about how the NHS is resourced in each devolved country. The total expenditure on the NHS across the UK was approximately £61 billion for 1999/2000. At just under 6.9% of gross domestic product (GDP) this figure is low in comparison with the amount of public money spent on health care in other countries (see Chapter 1).

The NHS today

SECRETARY OF STATE/DEPARTMENT OF HEALTH

Key posts and structures

The secretary of state for health has legal responsibility for promoting a comprehensive health service, dating from the NHS Acts of 1946 and 1977. He or she heads a team of ministers and parliamentary under-secretaries (junior ministers) who are drawn from the governing party and selected by the prime minister. Each member of the team has responsibility for particular aspects of the NHS, for example for public health.

In Scotland, Northern Ireland and Wales, equivalent ministerial roles exist following the establishment of the Scottish Parliament and Welsh and Northern Ireland Assemblies.

Policy and direction

The structure, priorities and, indeed, future of the NHS are all matters for political debate. Health issues rank highly among voters' concerns at election time. There are marked differences in political opinions on the health service between the major political parties. For example, the approach of Conservative governments in recent years was characterised as putting the NHS on a business footing, with the separation of 'purchaser' and 'provider' and the introduction of an 'internal market' (see Chapter 1). Great emphasis was placed by Conservative governments on efficiency and throughput. This differs from the current (as we write in December 2000) Labour government's stated collaborative approach of moving to 'integrated' care, with an emphasis on the quality as well as quantity of services, although different terminology is used. For example, 'throughput' now tends to be labelled 'access', and includes, for example, waiting lists and waiting times as key issues.

The secretary of state for health is responsible for the overall direction of travel for the NHS, making policy decisions and determining how best to spend the allocated budget. The constraints on the secretary of state are financial, dependent on the Treasury allocation of money, and political, dependent on the prime minister's favour and the agreement of his or her cabinet colleagues. The prime minister appoints and may remove the secretary of state. Important policy changes are agreed by the

Cabinet which then sets out the overall framework and principles by which government policy is guided. The secretary of state sets out policy in White and Green Papers as well as in statements and speeches throughout the year. The Department of Health also issued guidance on priorities and planning on an annual basis, but these are now issued as *joint* guidance for the NHS and social service departments, as part of the government's commitment to a seamless service for the end user, i.e. the patient or client.

Accountability to Parliament

The secretary of state and his or her team are held accountable for their actions to the Westminster Parliament in a number of ways. Convention dictates that any major changes to the health service should be explained to Parliament through statements or questions in the House. Any MP may probe the work of the secretary of state through oral questions (each secretary of state in turn being called to the despatch box) or by submitting written questions.

More fundamental changes, such as the removal of the internal market and its replacement with 'integrated care', are described in Green (consultation) or White Papers and presented to the House. These may be debated at greater length. White Papers such as those introducing the 'new NHS' usually precede legislation and both Houses of Parliament scrutinise and debate draft legislation (bills) in detail before they reach the statute book and become law. The legislation to end the internal market is contained in The Health Act which received Royal Assent in June 1999 (Department of Health 1999b).

Other means of scrutiny are also available to MP's – for example through the select committee system within which more detailed inquiries on particular subjects are undertaken. These may be influential in altering government policy (for example the recommendations contained in 'Changing Childbirth' (Department of Health 1993) followed the House of Commons Health Committee report on maternity services). Other statutory bodies are also held accountable by Parliament. For example, the health services ombudsman (the parliamentary commissioner for administration) presents a report to the House which is then scrutinised by the Select Committee on Public Administration.

How effective is such scrutiny? On the one hand it may be argued that any effective scrutiny of health policy is lost in the

The NHS today

battle to score party political points. This may be particularly true as we write, as a general election must be held within the next 16 months. Question time in the House of Commons rarely elicits any meaningful debate on the direction of travel for the NHS. On the other hand, the requirement to justify and explain actions taken is vital in a democracy in which MPs are the 'people's representatives'.

The government has power to remove NHS Trust/Health Authority chairs and non-executive directors, and has powers to intervene if the quality of services is unsatisfactory. This power of intervention will be explored later in the chapter where the role of the Commission for Health Improvement is discussed.

NHS EXECUTIVE

Key posts and structure

The NHS Executive (NHSE) is part of the Department of Health (Fig. 2.1). Its role is to provide support to ministers and to provide leadership and management functions to NHS commissioners and providers.

The NHSE has offices in London and Leeds and eight regional offices across England. Staff employed in the NHSE and its regional offices are civil servants. The regional offices assumed greater importance with the abolition of Regional Health Authorities in 1995.

It is worthy of note that the government is strengthening the connection between Department of Health policy and the NHS Executive. The recent appointment of Nigel Crisp as the Chief Executive of the NHS in England *and* as a Permanent Secretary reinforces this relationship.

The regional offices, along with regional directors of public health, oversee the work of the NHS locally. Arrangements for Wales, Scotland and Northern Ireland are addressed later.

Implementation of policy

The NHS Executive regional offices in England have an important role to play in ensuring that partnership becomes a reality in the new NHS. They will make sure that Health Authorities and Primary Care Groups work together, particularly in making

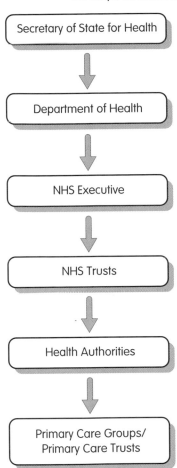

Figure 2.1 The structure of the NHS.

arrangements for commissioning specialist health services at a regional level. They will also ensure that local partnerships are developed between the NHS and local authorities.

Regional distribution of funding

Resources are allocated to Health Authorities and Primary Care Groups/Trusts according to a national formula which takes into account the different needs of local populations. Since devolution, some inconsistencies have emerged between the funding allocation of the four countries which will be addressed.

The NHS today

Performance measurement

The NHSE in England, the NHS Directorate in Wales, the NHS Management Executive in Scotland and the Health and Personal Services Management Group in Northern Ireland will attempt to maximise the performance of Health Authorities/Health Boards, monitoring their work and holding them to account. A 'carrot and stick' approach is proposed. Good progress will reap financial rewards for those authorities which do well against their Health Improvement Programme (HImP) (see below) targets and objectives. Health Improvement Programmes are action programmes led by Health Authorities and Health Boards, but involving NHS Trusts, Primary Care Groups/Local Health Groups/Local Health Care Cooperatives and others, to improve local health and health care. The reward will be non-recurrent funding for local projects in support of Health Improvement Programmes. They will also closely monitor poor progress, offering targeted management support, and may intervene as a final resort to demand leadership or managerial changes.

The NHS Plan in England introduces a notion of 'earned autonomy' (Department of Health 2000, paragraph 6.25) which encourages the devolving of decision making to local level as organisations become more successful in achieving their standards. This follows on from the emphasis in the 'new NHS' of giving the responsibility of shaping and commissioning care to clinical professionals working in the community. All NHS organisations will be assessed against the Performance Assessment Framework and will (publicly) every year be classified as 'green', 'yellow' or 'red'. Red organisations are those which are failing to meet a number of core national targets. Green organisations will be meeting all the core national targets, and in addition, will score in the top 25% of organisations against the Performance Assessment Framework. Yellow organisations will meet all core national targets, but may not make the top 25% within the Performance Assessment Framework. The criteria will be set nationally. However the assessment will be carried out by regional offices, and the Commission for Health Improvement (see later in this chapter) will act as an independent verifier of performance.

National Service Frameworks

In order to improve the consistency of standards of service across England and Wales, the new NHS requires the development of

The broad context of health care

National Service Frameworks (NSFs). Frameworks are to be based on particular areas of care and those for mental health and coronary heart disease are already issued. A National Service Framework for older people is to be issued imminently as this book goes to press. These frameworks will attempt to determine the best way of providing particular services, for example, what kinds of care are best delivered at primary, secondary or tertiary level care as emerged following the 'Calman–Hine' model of cancer services. This recommended that cancer services should be organised in three levels from primary care, to local hospitals, to larger centres where less common cancers could be treated and services such as radiotherapy could be provided.

Clinical governance

The new NHS requires Trusts to undertake a new form of accountability known as clinical governance. Trusts are under a duty to provide quality services. Clinical governance builds on the principles of corporate governance. It means that chief executives *personally* carry ultimate responsibility for the quality of services as well as the proper use of resources.

Chief executives are required to ensure that local arrangements are in place to fulfil the new duties regarding quality of service. 'The New NHS: Modern, Dependable' (Department of Health 1997) and sister White Papers identify the need for arrangements to include:

- action to ensure that risks are avoided;
- action to ensure that adverse events are rapidly detected, openly investigated and lessons learned; and
- action to ensure that good practice is rapidly disseminated and systems are in place to ensure continuous improvements in clinical care.

To achieve this Trusts have established a subcommittee of the Trust Board, led by a Board member, usually the Chief Nurse or Medical Director, that has responsibility for ensuring the internal clinical governance. Monthly reports are required and an annual quality report must be produced.

There are two key principles which underpin clinical governance. First, the principle that all clinical professionals should have a much greater say in how resources are spent. Second, the principle that quality issues are not solely the responsibility of the clinical professionals: quality is a whole organisation

The NHS today

41

responsibility. The aim is to ensure that clinicians and managers work in partnership to improve the quality of services. Thus clinical professionals need to develop their management acumen in the same way in which managers need to develop an understanding of clinical need.

HEALTH AUTHORITIES AND BOARDS

Structure

In December 1999 there were 99 Health Authorities in England and five in Wales. In Scotland there were 15 Health Boards. In Northern Ireland, four joint Health and Social Services Boards operate within an integrated Department of Health and Social Services.

Health Authorities comprise a chair plus a board of executive and non-executive directors who work together to formulate strategy and monitor performance. The chief executive, along with the other executive directors, is responsible for the day-to-day running of the authority. Executive directors are experts, each with their own functional responsibilities. Important decisions are taken by the whole board, thus allowing non-executive directors (often with expertise from outside the health services) to play an important role. Changes proposed in 'The New NHS' mean that local authority chief executives participate in meetings of Health Authorities. This change is to ensure that local authorities and Health Authorities work more closely together, particularly in the production and implementation of Health Improvement Programmes.

The primary function of Health Authorities is changing. Health Authorities in England emerged in 1996 as a result of the merger of District Health Authorities (DHAs) and Family Health Service Authorities (FHSAs). Up to April 1999 Health Authorities, along with GP fundholders (which were abolished by The Health Act 1999, except in Northern Ireland where fundholding continues until April 2001), commissioned health services for their local population. This changed as the Primary Care Groups (PCGs) and the Primary Care Trusts (PCTs) emerged in England in April 1999 and April 2000 respectively.

At present Health Authorities take on a more strategic commissioning role, and act a point of reference for the newer Primary Care organisations. It is not clear what role the Health

The broad context of health care

Authorities will take in the future, but it is likely that they will be small in size, and strategic rather than operational in focus.

Similarly, Local Health Groups (LHGs) provide primary services in Wales, and Local Health Care Cooperatives in Scotland. These differences are explored further later in this chapter.

Primary Care Groups were proposed in the English White Paper (Department of Health 1998). PCGs came into action in April 1999 and brought together doctors and nurses and other professionals in order to commission both primary care and hospital services for their local populations. The legislation allows for PCGs to mature into Primary Care Trusts (PCTs) and the first of these took on PCT status in April 2000.

In England four options for primary care were outlined. These are:

1. Level 1 – a PCG supporting/advising a Health Authority in its commissioning role
2. Level 2 – a PCG taking devolved responsibility for managing the budget
3. Level 3 – a PCT commissioning hospital and community services for its population
4. Level 4 – a PCT which, in addition to level 3 responsibilities, can provide community services for the population and can employ staff and manage facilities in its own right.

The NHS Plan requires that all PCGs become PCTs by April 2004. Parallel in England, from The NHS Plan will emerge new *Care Trusts* which will be Primary Care Trusts (PCTs) with the addition of social services, thus bringing the NHS and social services together with new agreements to pool resources. These Care Trusts will commission health and social care as a single activity, and will be particularly beneficial to older people by facilitating the packages to help them remain at home for longer.

'The New NHS' (Department of Health 1997) proposed that Health Authorities should delegate their commissioning function to Primary Care Groups (see below). As a result it is anticipated that there will be fewer Health Authorities covering larger areas. However, the changes will take place over a period of years. Some commissioning, such as that required for special-ist services, will remain at Health Authority level, or, for some services such as renal, commissioning will occur at regional or subregional level by groups of Health Authorities.

Health Authorities are to be placed under two new statutory duties: first to work in partnership with the NHS and other local bodies; and second to improve the health of their populations.

The NHS today

The statutory nature of these new duties (i.e. enshrined in an Act of Parliament) demonstrates the value which is placed in the new NHS on partnership working and addressing quality issues. They also fulfil a range of other functions such as regulation and inspection of nursing homes, and this function too is moving towards a joint function with the local authority, who currently have the responsibility for inspecting residential homes.

In Wales, Health Authorities will develop along very similar lines to the English Health Authorities but a reduction in their number is not anticipated. Local Health Groups are subcommittees of the Health Authority, rather than independent bodies, thus there are no primary health care trusts in Wales. Arrangements in Wales are discussed in more detail in Application 2.3.

In Scotland, Primary Care Trusts were established in April 1999 and have responsibility for all primary and community care, including services for learning disabilities and mental health. Local Health Care Cooperatives focus on developing provision of services, and have no commissioning role.

Strategic leadership

Fewer, leaner Health Authorities will be able to provide 'strategic leadership' to their local health services. In particular, they will lead the development of Health Improvement Programmes, identifying local health and health care needs and determining which services are needed to meet these needs. 'The New NHS' identifies seven key tasks for Health Authorities in the new NHS (Box 2.2). The first four of these tasks reflect Health Authorities' responsibilities prior to April 1999. However, as they lose their commissioning function, the government anticipates that Health Authorities will place a stronger focus on public health issues.

Box 2.2   Seven key tasks for Health Authorities in the new NHS

1. To assess health needs
2. To draw up Health Improvement Programmes, in partnership with others
3. To decide the range and location of health services
4. To determine local standards and targets
5. To support the development of Primary Care Groups
6. To allocate resources to Primary Care Groups
7. To hold Primary Care Groups to account

The broad context of health care

Public health

The public health functions of Health Authorities are already well developed and include health surveillance, control of communicable diseases, assessment of health needs, monitoring of health outcomes, and evaluating the health impact of local plans and developments. Public health is given a new emphasis in the NHS, particularly with the publication of three Green Papers with the specific aim of improving public health (Department of Health 1998, Scottish Office Department of Health 1998, Welsh Office Department of Health 1998a), and the subsequent White Papers, 'Our Healthier Nation: a Contract for Health' (Department of Health 1998) for England, 'Towards a Healthier Scotland' (Scottish Office Department of Health 1999) for Scotland and 'Better Health – Better Wales' (Welsh Office 1998b) for Wales.

Health Improvement Programmes

Health Improvement Programmes (HImPs) are the means by which Health Authorities and, in Scotland, Health Boards and others fulfil their duty to improve the health of their local populations. Health Authorities and Boards will lead local alliances to develop HImPs. These look at the overall health needs of the local population and the health care requirements. HImPs set out how the national contracts for health are to be delivered locally, and set local priorities and targets, focusing action on those who need the most support. They establish the range, location and investment needed in local health services. HImPs focus on how the NHS and other local bodies will work together to achieve specific targets to improve public health and health care.

HImPs in England are 3-year programmes (started in April 1999), with parts being reviewed each year. Similarly in Wales a 3-year agenda has been set, with broad intentions for years 4 and 5 outlined. In Scotland, HImPs will be a 5-year rolling programme.

Setting local targets and monitoring

Health Authorities/Boards will monitor the implementation of HImPs. Annual accountability agreements will be made between Health Authorities/Boards and relevant primary care organisations in each country to set key objectives and targets for improving health and health care. Health Authorities/Boards will also be given reserve powers to ensure that major investment

The NHS today

decisions, such as capital development or new consultant appointments, are consistent with the local HImP.

Overseeing the development of Primary Care Groups, including allocating resources and accountability

Health Authorities in England had the task of ensuring that Primary Care Groups (PCGs) were established in their area. The actual configuration of such groups was determined from 'bottom-up', following local discussions between all interested players. The population size for each group is circa 100 000. The Health Authority's role was to ensure that the discussions took place, and to notify the NHS Executive of the local configuration.

Health Authorities are responsible for allocating resources to PCGs. 'The New NHS' proposed that the budgets for hospital and community services, prescribing and GP infrastructure should be merged into one funding stream. The whole budget is cash limited and the formula for allocating both primary and secondary resources has been addressed.

Health Authorities are also charged with resolving any disagreements between Primary Care Trusts and NHS Trusts.

Health Action Zones

Health Authorities have an important role in communicating with and involving local people in decisions about local services. One way in which new means of communicating and developing partnerships can be explored is through Health Action Zones (HAZs).

Twenty-six HAZs have been established by the government in England in areas of deprivation and poor health to tackle health inequalities and modernise services through local innovation. Although the HAZ communities vary significantly in their characteristics, they face common problems of ill health and disadvantage. HAZs represent areas of the country with some of the highest levels of deprivation and the poorest levels of health.

HAZs are partnerships between the NHS, local authorities, the voluntary and private sectors, and community groups. The HAZ programmes represent a new approach to public health – linking health, regeneration, employment, education, housing and anti-poverty initiatives to respond to the needs of vulnerable groups and deprived communities. The principles on which

The broad context of health care

HAZs are based include partnership working, involvement of local people and involvement of front-line staff.

Health Authorities are given a key role in drawing together all the local players, including the public, and ensuring that they work together. However, Health Authorities remain indirectly accountable to the public they serve.

An example of how specific health needs are being met in Scotland is discussed in Application 2.1.

NHS TRUSTS

Structure

Self-governing hospital or community trusts were established under the NHS and Community Care Act 1990, and the first wave of trusts went 'live' in April 1991. Under the new NHS in England and Wales, NHS Trusts remain responsible locally for operational management and for the employment of staff. They will continue to be run by boards of executive and non-executive directors, and the chief executive officer is personally accountable to the secretary of state for the business of the Trust.

In Scotland, Trusts are managed by a trust team led by a part-time non-executive chairman appointed by the secretary of state. The chairman sits ex-officio as a non-executive member of their local Health Board, reflecting the closer integration of Health Boards and Trusts in Scotland.

There are two types of Trust in Scotland: Primary Care Trusts (responsible for primary, community and mental health services) and Acute Hospital Trusts. The government intends that there should be only one Acute Hospital Trust in each Health Board although it is acknowledged that this may not be feasible in all areas. This has resulted in mergers occurring, as in England. The Scottish Plan was published in December 2000 and suggests some radical changes including abolishing Trusts. The implementation guidance is likely to be available in early 2001.

In England many NHS Trusts have undergone reconfiguration or merger in order to achieve financial savings, whilst maintaining quality of provision. The spirit of the White Paper insists that this should be driven by the best interests of the patient, yet this has yet to be established in financial terms, as early experiences suggest that fewer savings are to be made than was assumed.

In Wales, mergers have resulted in the establishment of 16 Trusts, the majority of these being integrated Trusts, providing acute, community and mental health services.

The NHS today

Strategy and planning

NHS Trusts will be placed under a statutory duty to work in partnership with other NHS bodies. The Health Act (Department of Health 1999b) reinforces this. The new NHS proposes a system of 'integrated care' where Trusts cooperate and share information rather than compete. Trusts will have a new role to play in shaping the local Health Improvement Programmes with other stakeholders.

NHS Trusts will continue to have an important role in determining workforce requirements. Working with local education consortia, NHS Trusts along with other groups calculate their likely need for personnel (for example, the number of nurses required) and the likely educational requirements. Consortia are to be replaced by workforce confederations in 2001. These organisations will take the lead in developing the workforce to ensure an appropriate staff pool for the healthcare needs of the population. Regional Education and Development Groups (REDGs) then advise regional offices of the NHSE on the coherence of the local workforce planning and on the direction of education and training. This system is set up to ensure that education planning at national level responds to the needs of the NHS at local level, and plans for service developments. In Scotland, Trust Implementation Plans will be prepared by each NHS Trust, in agreement with their local Health Board, setting out how the Trust will deliver the Health Improvement Programme.

Operational management

NHS Trusts in England are accountable to their local NHSE regional office for fulfilling their statutory duties. They are accountable to Health Authorities and Primary Care Groups for the services they deliver. The annual system of contracting for services between NHS Trusts as providers of services and the PCGs/PCTs as commissioners has been replaced by 'service agreements' of 3 years or more as fundholder status is abolished, along with the internal market as a result of The Health Act (Department of Health 1999b). The service agreements place a greater emphasis on the patient as the centre of care delivery, and service agreements are thus being designed to mirror this focus by incorporating processes such as patient journeys, clinical pathways, etc. The service agreements will also include explicit standards for quality and efficiency.

All NHS Trusts are required to publish the prices they charge for treatments and services to allow benchmarking and comparison between Trusts. A National Schedule of Reference Costs will be drawn up to improve the ability of commissioners and providers to compare costs and efficiency. Commissioners will be able to question providers who propose higher than average charges. Thus comparison, rather than competition, between Trusts intends to achieve efficiency and value for money.

Health Authorities, PCGs/PCTs and Trusts are required to publish details of their performance measured against a National Performance Framework. This will allow comparisons between Trusts in six areas of performance:

- health improvement in the local population
- fair access to services
- effective delivery of health care
- value for money
- experience of patients and carers
- health outcomes.

In Scotland, the Trust Implementation Plan will be the means by which the Trust is held accountable to the Health Board. Trusts are required to publish a range of clinical performance indicators, to demonstrate the effectiveness of their care. This of course may be changed as a result of the Scottish NHS Plan. However, currently there is nothing comparable to the English 'service agreements'. Instead, Acute Hospital Trusts and Primary Care Trusts are to set up joint planning and budgeting arrangements to cover the interface between primary, secondary and tertiary care. The Health Board, through the Trust Implementation Plan, will set out the resources it intends to make available to that individual Trust. The Health Board will also establish a Joint Investment Fund for the interface plans. The new guidance due in the early part of 2001 will clarify this further.

PRIMARY CARE GROUPS, LOCAL HEALTH GROUPS, LOCAL HEALTH CARE COOPERATIVES AND PRIMARY CARE TRUSTS

Whilst maintaining the underlying principles, different models have emerged in the four UK countries. In England, Primary Care Groups and Trusts have been established. In Wales Local Health Groups parallel the English Primary Care Groups but

The NHS today

remain as subcommittees of Health Authorities rather than becoming free-standing bodies. In Scotland, Local Health Care Cooperatives are the nearest parallel but will have no commissioning function. Instead they will be brought together with other providers of primary and community services to form Primary Care Trusts.

Two possible models are currently under discussion in Northern Ireland (in the consultation paper 'Fit for the Future'; DHSS 1998). Model A is very similar to the English model, with Health and Social Service Boards fulfilling a similar function to that of Health Authorities, and with the presence of Primary Care Groups and Health and Social Services Trusts. Model B is a radical departure. It proposes Local Care Agencies to replace Health and Social Services Boards and some or all Trusts. Local Care Agencies would have both a commissioner and provider function, though the two would be kept separate. Primary Care Partnerships within Local Care Agencies would commission most health care. This is investigated further in Application 2.2.

England

Structure of Primary Care Groups and Primary Care Trusts

Primary Care Groups and Trusts are the commissioning bodies in the new NHS. Prior to their establishment, there was a great variety in patterns of commissioning. In some areas GP fundholders covered large parts of the population and commissioned services on their behalf. In other areas the presence of GP fundholders was small and most of the commissioning fell to Health Authorities. There was also a range of other schemes such as Total Purchasing Projects and Locality Commissioning Groups where non-fundholding GPs worked closely with their Health Authorities to commission care for their patients.

The new NHS aims to ensure that there is greater consistency in the pattern of commissioning. GP fundholding has been criticised as leading to inequity: patients of fundholders were said to have had an unfair advantage over those of non-fundholders as the former had greater flexibility over referral to secondary care providers. The Health Act 1999 abolished GP fundholding and now all general practitioners are part of the new PCGs or PCTs.

Nevertheless, the new NHS aims to build on the progress that has been made in involving GPs in determining the pattern of service for their patients. Under a 'primary-care led NHS', it makes sense to put those who have the most contact with patients – GPs, practice nurses and community nurses – in the driving seat for commissioning, and this was the principle behind the establishment of Primary Care Groups and Trusts. PCGs/PCTs bring together all the GPs and community nurses in a particular area, along with other players, such as social services, to commission both primary and secondary services for their local populations.

The new NHS is specific about the strengthened role which is envisaged for nurses working in all areas of the community. The governing body of the PCG/PCT must include nursing staff and social services as well as GPs drawn from the area. Nurses are to be involved in both the strategic and operational functions of the new group, and one or two nurses will be included on the PCG/PCT Board. This of course places responsibilities upon the nurses to develop their management skills. Level 4 PCTs will be able to employ staff, and thus community nurses/midwives will be employed by those organisations rather than the Community or Acute Trust. The structure of the PCT Boards broadly mirrors those of other Trusts (see earlier in the chapter).

Primary Care Groups/Trusts have developed 'around natural communities' serving a population of about 100 000 people. In most cases the Groups/Trusts are coterminous with local social services boundaries to encourage the delivery of seamless patient care.

Commissioning local services (different models)

The White Paper for England (Department of Health 1998) set out four stages of Primary Care Group/Trust, depending on local circumstances and the extent to which GPs were already involved in commissioning in a particular area. First stage PCGs ensure that GPs and nurses play an advisory role to their Health Authority. Second stage PCGs take devolved responsibility for managing the budget for health care, but the Health Authority will retain overall financial responsibility. The third stage PCT is a free-standing body, accountable to the Health Authority for commissioning care. The fourth stage PCT can take on the additional responsibility of providing community health services (thus blurring the distinction between commissioner and provider). The government intends all PCGs to progress along this path to assume fuller responsibilities over time, and The Health Act 1999 allowed the first wave of Primary Care Trusts to come into existence on 1 April 2000 in England and Wales. In Scotland all PCTs were established in April 1999. The NHS Plan intends that all PCGs have converted to PCTs by April 2004.

A stage four Primary Care Trust will be able to provide community health services – including community hospitals – and these may merge with an existing community NHS Trust in time. Primary Care Trusts will not provide acute services, nor are they expected to take responsibility for specialist mental health or learning disability services. The government's preference is for specialist mental health or learning disability Trusts to be established in order that an integrated range of services from community to hospital care can be provided. The new Care Trusts will be able to commission seamless packages of care spanning the traditional NHS/local authority roles.

The PCG/PCTs, rather than the individual medical practices, will reach service agreements with NHS Trusts.

Some specialist services, such as bone marrow transplant, continue to serve the population of more than one Health Authority. Responsibility for commissioning specialist hospital services which need a national focus falls to the National Specialist Commissioning Advisory Group and the High Secure Psychiatric Services Commissioning Board. Regional offices have responsibility for ensuring effective commissioning of services which fall between national and Health Authority level.

Involvement in health improvement programmes

The main functions of PCGs/PCTs in relation to health improvement, as set out in the White Paper, are to:

- contribute to the Health Authority's Health Improvement Programme,
- promote the health of the local population,
- commission health services,
- monitor performance against service agreements they have with NHS Trusts,
- develop primary care, and
- better integrate primary and community health services and work more closely with social services.

The government is clear that there are two main aims for PCGs/PCTs: to act as the new commissioners and to improve the health of the population they serve by reducing inequalities in service provision.

Clinical governance and quality issues

The principle of clinical governance is applied in primary care. Each PCG/PCT must nominate a senior professional to take the lead on standards generally and on professional development within the PCG or PCT.

Individual practices within the PCG/PCT are encouraged to identify an individual to take the lead responsibility but it is recognised that in small practices this may not be possible. Primary Care Groups/Trusts are expected to reach service agreements with providers which reflect the views of all the members. However, PCGs/PCTs will bring together a wide variety of interests, including both ex-fundholding and ex-non-fundholding GPs, nurses, social services, Health Authority non-executives, and lay members. Unanimity may not be easy to achieve amongst diverse groups, unused to cooperative ways of working. The dynamics of the PCG/PCT may be influenced profoundly by their position on the PCG ladder, from advisory subcommittee of the Health Authority, to free-standing Primary Care Trust. Much will depend on where commissioning expertise lies locally. PCGs may prefer to start slowly, taking on more responsibility over time, or they may wish to exert their independence from Health Authorities as soon as possible by working towards PCT status as soon as possible.

Wales

In Wales, Local Health Groups fulfil the same functions as the English Primary Care Groups, commissioning services for their local populations. The emphasis is again on the inclusive nature of Local Health Groups. The governing body of the Local Health Group includes GPs, other community health professionals, social services and other community interests such as the voluntary sector.

The key difference between PCGs in England and Local Health Groups is that the latter remain as subcommittees of their Health Authorities. Although Local Health Groups have access to budgets for hospital and community health services, the actual flow of funds is between Health Authority and Trust. Local Health Groups work with Health Authorities to monitor the performance of NHS Trusts in Wales. In situations where quality standards fail in Trusts, the Welsh Assembly will have power to intervene. Application 2.3 expands further upon the Welsh perspective.

The NHS today

Primary care in Scotland currently is organised in Primary Care Trusts (PCTs), one of two types of Trust. As in the English Primary Care Trusts, these organisations bring together general practice with community services. Unlike England, Primary Care Trusts currently may manage services for people with learning disabilities or people with mental illness. PCTs are responsible for formulating primary care policy and supporting general practitioners, and for developing integrated primary care. They work in partnership with Health Boards and Acute Hospital Trusts to deliver the Health Improvement Programme. Primary Care Trusts were established throughout Scotland in April 1999.

General practice is more strongly coordinated through the formation of Local Health Care Cooperatives. Local Health Care Cooperatives are networks of general practices with responsibility for managing and delivering services across a defined area based on natural communities, which may vary according to geography, in the population range 25 000 to 150 000.

While the importance of the extended general practice team is recognised in the Scottish White Paper (Scottish Office Department of Health 1998), the lead in primary care is clearly given to the general practitioner. Primary Care Trusts receive funding from their Health Boards. In turn, PCTs allocate resources to their local Cooperatives. Cooperatives are responsible for managing and operating their budgets but the actual cash is be administered by the PCT, to whom the Cooperatives will be financially accountable.

However, the Scottish NHS Plan intends to change this framework by abolishing Trusts. More detail is not available at the time of writing, and it is anticipated that guidance will be published in early 2001.

Commission for Health Improvement

The Commission for Health Improvement (CHI) is a national body, proposed in the 'The New NHS' to oversee the quality of clinical services within a framework of clinical governance. Consideration is being given to whether this model may be extended to Northern Ireland. The NHS in Wales will be involved in the establishment of CHI. Scotland already has a range of different bodies to oversee quality. The Commission has been compared with a national inspectorate for health services,

The broad context of health care

undertaking a rolling programme of inspections of all health bodies to ensure that minimum standards are reached.

The Commission also has a quality assurance role, monitoring and overseeing clinical quality systems. Working at arm's length from the government, the membership of the Commission is drawn from the professions, NHS, academic and patient representatives. The Commission may be called in by Health Authorities, Primary Care Groups or NHS Trusts, or may intervene on the direction of the secretary of state where the quality of services is unsatisfactory. In the first instance, the Commission will work with the local health organisation, but if local solutions are insufficient, the Commission may recommend other action to the secretary of state.

The Commission for Health Improvement (CHI) aims to address two major principles in the new NHS: achieving greater national consistency in the quality of care, and improving performance, working alongside the National Institute for Clinical Excellence. However, there are concerns as to whether the two potential functions of the CHI – supporting the introduction of quality systems and inspecting standards of service – are compatible within one organisation. As we write, this relationship is now under debate. We have already seen a number of organisations being brought to task over poor quality services by the CHI, and this appears set to continue.

'The New NHS: Modern Dependable' (Department of Health 1997) suggests that the Commission may also conduct systematic service reviews, ensuring implementation of the National Service Frameworks (NSFs) and the guidelines developed by the National Institute for Clinical Excellence (NICE), a body set up to promote clinical and cost effectiveness and to disseminate clinical guidelines.

National Institute for Clinical Excellence (NICE)

This body has been established to improve the dissemination of good practice in England and Wales. NICE produces guidelines based on available evidence of what is clinically and cost effective. It disseminates clinical guidelines and examples of good practice in clinical audit. The membership of NICE is drawn from the NHS, health professions, health economists, patients and academics.

In Scotland, a very different model is emerging. Scotland is already far advanced in its promotion of clinical effectiveness. 'Designed to Care' (Scottish Office Department of Health 1997) promises a review of the various organisations and initiatives involved in promoting quality. These include the Clinical Resource and Audit Group (CRAG), the Scottish Health Purchasing Information Centre (SHPIC) and the Scottish Needs Assessment Programme (SNAP). The aim is to produce a nationally organised process of quality assurance, building on the work already underway, but delivering it in a more coordinated fashion. The Scottish Health Technology Assessment Centre (SHTAC) evaluates the cost effectiveness of innovations in health care, including new drugs.

The NHS Plan

This important document was published by the Department of Health in July 2000 and is to be the driving force to see through the radical changes in health care delivery for the twenty-first century. The structures discussed above are there to support these changes, but real difference in quality is achieved not by altering organisational structure and job roles, nor by putting in further resource. Quality is achieved by engaging the staff in teamwork to deliver care. To do this effectively clinical staff need to understand how policy affects practice, and how they, at the sharp end, can influence strategic decision making, and thus achieve best value for money. The NHS Plan refers specifically to England, but as we send this book to press, the Scottish Plan has been published (December 2000), although implementation guidance will not be available until early in 2001. We are aware that similar documents for the other two countries are imminent.

The NHS Plan for England can be accessed on the internet: www.nhs.uk/nhsplan

The NHS Plan for Scotland can be accessed on the internet: www.scotland.gov.uk/library3/health/onh-00.asp

SUMMARY

It is interesting to consider whether in the long term the new structure will achieve the principles set for the new NHS. In the total UK picture, greater consistency within the four nations, for example through the introduction of NICE and National Service Frameworks, is tempered by greater differences between them. For example, it might be argued that the Scottish model is more radical than that for England in its attempt to abolish the internal market.

The broad context of health care

Local responsibility for care is delivered through Primary Care Groups/Trusts, and eventually Care Trusts and their equivalents, based on the needs and priorities of local communities and operating within locally agreed Health Improvement Programmes.

Quality and partnership are the watchwords of the new NHS. Quality is being managed in a variety of ways, from the introduction of NICE and CHI and their equivalents, to the new statutory duties placed on NHS bodies and the introduction of clinical governance. Partnership are made compulsory by The Health Act 1999 as the language of 'contracting' and 'competition' is replaced by 'service agreements' and 'integrated care'. Partnership is to facilitate the use of benchmarking and comparison between Trusts, which, along with the CHI and the 'carrot and stick' approach adopted by NHSE, should lead to the improvement of efficiency and performance. All these issues will be rolled out by The NHS Plan in the respective countries.

References

Department of Health (1993) Changing childbirth, London: HMSO.

Department of Health (1997) The new NHS: modern, dependable. London: The Stationery Office.

Department of Health (1998) Our healthier nation: – a contract for health. London: The Stationery Office.

Department of Health (1999a) Saving lives: our healthier nation. London: The Stationery Office.

Department of Health (1999b) The Health Act. London: The Stationery Office.

Department of Health (2000) The NHS Plan. London: The Stationery Office.

DHSS (1998) Fit for the future. A consultation document on the government's proposals for the future of the Health and Personal Social Services in Northern Ireland. Belfast: DHSS.

Scottish Office Department of Health (1997) Designed to care – renewing the National Health Service in Scotland. Edinburgh: The Stationery Office.

Scottish Office Department of Health (1998) Working together for a healthier Scotland. Edinburgh: The Stationery Office.

Scottish Office Department of Health (1999) Towards a healthier Scotland. Edinburgh: The Stationery Office.

Scottish Office Department of Health (2000) The NHS Plan. Edinburgh: The Stationery Office.

Welsh Office (1998a) NHS Wales – putting patients first. Cardiff: The Stationery Office.

Welsh Office (1998b) Better health – better Wales: a consultation paper. London: The Stationery Office.

The NHS today

Application 2:1 *Sue Williams*

Managing health and social services in Scotland

In this case study, Sue Williams outlines the rationale for the introduction of social inclusion partnerships (SIPs) in Scotland, and points out the key issues in ensuring their success: partnership working, and meeting real needs, as defined by the people of the neighbourhood. You will read more about joint working practices in Chapter 3.

Glasgow has 10 of the most deprived areas in the United Kingdom, and it has been recognised that despite real improvements, Scotland's record of ill health remains a serious concern. Tackling this ill health is not just about providing efficient, effective health services but is also about investing in initiatives that will bring about good health. There are inequalities in health between various social groups, and between geographical areas. A coherent and coordinated programme to tackle the issue of poor health linked to housing, education, social inclusion and food safety is the only way to bring about a major change in health status. The health service has therefore a crucial role in the development of social inclusion partnerships.

During the late 1990s when the Scottish government was considering the issues of social inclusion, it noted that the problems associated with social exclusion were very complex. It was recognised that there was a complex set of linked problems including unemployment, poor skills, low income, poor housing, high crime levels, bad health and family breakdown. The government identified the long-term objective as developing ways of working which integrated programmes of action, not just at government level but at all levels, right through to local communities and neighbourhoods. It emphasised five key principles of promoting social inclusion: prevention, empowerment, inclusiveness, integration and understanding.

One of the key mechanisms in delivering these principles was to build stronger communities who would be able to advocate on behalf of the community and support those living within it. In 1998/99 social inclusion partnerships (SIPs) were formed and funded to encourage joint working between statutory and voluntary agencies and the community itself. SIPs aim to tackle the issue of social inclusion within the country's most deprived areas. Additional funding of £45 million was made available over a 3-year period to support the initiative.

The SIPs are to be established to take forward the regeneration of deprived communities, recognising that in no area of deprivation should they be left to deal with such complex problems without the support and commitment of all local agencies. A coordinated approach to exclusion is to be adopted which will tackle the problems from the perspective of the local people rather than from that of an individual agency. In particular, SIPs are expected to address the long-term prevention of social exclusion through work with children and their families.

Partnership working is encouraged to improve the quality of life and well being of those living in the area. The key characteristics of a SIP, as suggested by the Scottish Executive, are outlined in Box 2.1.1.

Partnership structures will be established formally for all SIPS and the health service is expected to take an active part. A significant message in the guidance distributed by the Scottish Executive was the need to re-orient mainstream

---

Box 2.1.1   Social inclusion partnerships: key characteristics

- They focus on the most needy members of society
- They coordinate and fill gaps between existing programmes to promote inclusion
- They seek to prevent people becoming socially excluded
- They have a significant emphasis on work with children and young people

Managing health and social services in Scotland

resources into and within the SIPs to gain improvements in local services.

It is not surprising, given the poor state of health and the levels of deprivation apparent in some parts of Glasgow, that funding would be directed to the proposals from the local agencies and voluntary groups to establish SIPs in the city. There were two possible approaches to formulating the proposals: one based on a geographical patch, and the second focused upon particular groups in the population, such as ethnic minorities. Seven proposals were accepted and agreed; a selection of those that were established are described below.

GEOGRAPHICAL SIPs

Greater Easterhouse

Population 37 500, Deprivation (Carstairs) Category 7.

This is an area in the east of the city consisting mainly of social housing built in the 1960s to replace the traditional Glasgow tenements in the city centre. The area had very little infrastructure, few amenities, high unemployment, and problems with substance abuse and drug addiction.

The Health Board already invests heavily in the area (around £21.9 million per annum), mostly on primary care. There is a health centre providing standard services such as general practitioners, health visitors, district nurses, community dentistry and a pharmacy, which is linked into the Methadone Programme. There is also a mental health resource centre providing outreach consultant clinics, psychology services and a team of community psychiatric nurses.

As part of the new initiative a health and well-being baseline study will be undertaken to inform future action and evaluation. There are plans to develop a health shop, to ensure the local population have access to clear information about health issues, and a safety scheme aimed at preventing childhood accidents both through information and the provision of safety equipment. The secondary school sited in the locality is a new 'community school' and will implement a range of health-related activities to meet the needs identified by both the staff and the local community. In particular they will focus on the emotional needs of pupils and of those who have poor school attendance.

A key issue for health in this area will be dealing with the problems arising from illegal drugs. The women in the community have already demonstrated their wish to eradicate drugs from their neighbourhood and make it a safe place for their children. There will be a need to work closely with other agencies both to provide appropriate services for those who are already drug users, and to develop new approaches that help to prevent the use of illegal drugs. A particular emphasis will be given to working with local schools and youth groups to ensure a clear unambiguous message is given about the dangers of substance abuse and illegal drugs in particular.

However, these measures on their own will not be successful unless adults in the community can see improvements in housing and greater job opportunities for themselves and their families, this is the challenge for the agencies working within in the SIP.

North Glasgow

Population 69 000, Deprivation (Carstairs) Category 7.

This includes areas to the north of the city centre such as Possilpark where again there is mostly social housing built in a more traditional tenement style. The area is run down, much of the older housing has been demolished, and re-development is in its early stages. The area has a health centre, a mental health resource centre, a centre dealing with drug problems and a nursing home has opened recently. There is a local shopping area but the goods are of poor quality and many of the premises have closed. There is also a local school and a community centre.

In this locality £45.3 million per annum has already been spent on health, including a budget of £60 000 dedicated to regeneration. Current priorities include joint work between housing and health to improve the environment, and a major oral health project aimed at the under-fives and primary school children to improve dentition. Breakfast clubs for school age children have been introduced to ensure that the school day starts with a healthy breakfast, as many children were arriving at school without having eaten.

Managing health and social services in Scotland

61

Additionally community fresh food shops have been established to ensure that the local population can purchase fresh fruit and vegetables at prices they are able to afford.

There will also be an investigation into the needs of older people and their carers, developing appropriate support tailored to meet the deficits identified by the exercise.

Whilst these initiatives go some way to ease the health problems of the locality, the agencies have to work closely with the community to improve the whole inclusion agenda.

Castlemilk

Population 18 000, Deprivation (Carstairs) Category 7.

In this area there has been a total health spend of £9 million. There is a modern health centre which houses one GP practice and community services. The GP practice draws 70% of its patients from the local area. A local health group already exists with a working action plan that includes:

- Training, employment and the local economy
- Housing issues
- Land use and the physical environment
- Social and community issues.

Defined objectives and targets have been developed for each issue. Local health priorities have been identified, and include prevention of accidents, community safety, services and support for young people, and care for people with special needs. Highlighted in this area is the issue of domestic violence, and policies related to women and women's health. In particular there will be an emphasis on young women living on a low income with smoking-related problems.

These three examples of geographical SIPs demonstrate the need for inclusive working between agencies to gain improvements in the well being of the population. They also highlight the considerable problems in relation to health and the need for the health service to be fully involved with the work of the partnerships. It is important to use the investment already available in a way that will empower the community to take charge of their own health.

SIPs TARGETED AT PARTICULAR GROUPS

Routes out of prostitution

This initiative aims to prevent further harm to individuals and also to secure social inclusion for these women. It will work by:

- preventing women, particularly young women/girls becoming involved in prostitution,
- providing viable alternatives for women who wish to stop prostituting and support them to take up safe housing, child care support, drug programmes, training and employment, and
- changing public and agency perceptions of prostitution.

  The proposal has three core components:

- A city-wide partnership that will develop and implement a strategic approach to the issues of prostitution.
- A small specialist intervention team to work with vulnerable girls and young women, providing support for those wishing to stop prostituting and make mainstream services more accessible.
- A review of all existing services provided by statutory agencies and voluntary organisations to ensure these services are more accessible and more responsive to need.

This will build upon the joint project funded by the Health Board and the city council that already provides a drop-in facility for these women with access to primary health care, needle exchange, and counselling and advocacy. It includes support for an escort service for women who need urgent hospital treatment, and free condoms for those attending the centre.

As can be seen from this example, a SIP that focuses on a particular client group can pull together all the resources that are currently available and redesign services to meet the identified needs of the group in a more appropriate way. It does not necessarily require additional resources, but certainly does require a fresh look at services and how they could provide an improved, integrated service.

Managing health and social services in Scotland

Managing health and social services in Northern Ireland

In this application, Bryans offers a brief overview of the way in which the changes in government have been applied in Northern Ireland, setting the scene by outlining how structures changed following the dissolution of the devolved Government. Bryans comments upon current thinking in relation to the delivery of quality health care in Northern Ireland, pointing out that there are particular challenges because of the political situation.

THE POLITICAL DIMENSION

Northern Ireland has a population of 1.6 million people, a large proportion of whom live in and around the City of Belfast, famous for both its heavy and light industries which include shipbuilding and aircraft manufacture. In health care terms, Belfast is the location for most of the regional centres of excellence and university campuses.

After the dissolution of the original devolved government in Northern Ireland, local government, which was provided through the traditional and familiar county, urban, and rural district council system, was dismantled with the local government restructuring in October 1973. This stripped out many major local government functions such as social services, community and public health, education, housing, environment, and placed them under the control of independently appointed organisations. Effectively, this means that elected representatives at local level had control of very few local services. Thus the delivery of both health and social services through integrated structures was an interesting and effective development which occurred as a result of this major change.

Some viewed this unified approach as being potentially cumbersome and threatening, but the advantages inherent in the facility for easier movement within the continuity of care spectrum and the flexibility of the management of resources to reflect changing patterns, have proved commendable. Indeed, they are structures that have survived the advent of general management, the internal market, care in the community, and the changes the evolution to trust status invoked.

However, the government's proposals for the reduction in health and social service bureaucracy as outlined in the paper 'Fit for the Future' (DHSS 1998) await the arrival of the local decision making process, through a devolved government. The re-establishment of more locally based democracy is seen as a desirable goal and is in keeping with present government policy.

The Belfast Agreement, sometimes called the 'Good Friday Agreement', achieved in 1998, was supported by the overwhelming majority of people both in Northern Ireland and in the Irish Republic, voting in simultaneous but separate referenda. Subsequently, the election by the people of Northern Ireland of a new 108 member legislative assembly was not followed by the formation of a power-sharing executive or cabinet. This failure was due mainly to fundamental differences of opinion of the interpretation of key issues in the Belfast Agreement, which for a time seemed to pose intractable difficulties.

However, after protracted and complex negotiations which were facilitated greatly by US Senator George Mitchell, an Executive has been formed and devolution of powers from Westminster was effected on 2 December 1999. In accordance with the terms of the Belfast Agreement, there are 10 ministers, a first minister and a deputy first minister in the Executive, but the total composition is divided equally between what is perceived to be the Roman Catholic and the Protestant communities.

The new minister for health, social services and public safety is Bairbre de Brun and she is 'pledged to tackle

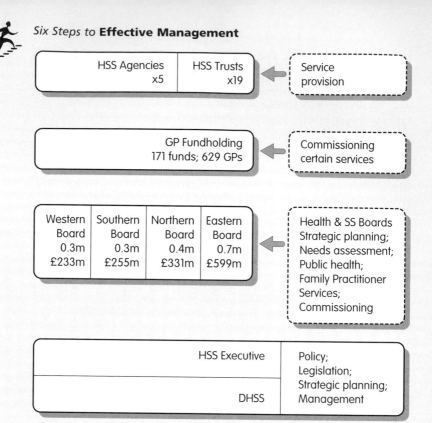

Figure 2.2.1 Current health and personal social services structure in Northern Ireland.

urgently the many issues that face the health and social services' (Executive Information Service 1999).

THE CURRENT SITUATION

The structure for the provision of health and personal social services to the people of Northern Ireland is illustrated in Figure 2.2.1. In some places, hospital and community health and personal social services are provided by one complex management entity. In other cases, particularly in conurbations where numbers appear to justify it, and there are recognised centres of excellence, hospital provision and community service provision are separate. The dominant consideration is said to be the protection of a 'seamless service', and professional interests are secured by ensuring that they are represented at all levels in the organisational

The broad context of health care

hierarchy. This variety of organisational provision manifests good examples of the application of the theory of business planning and management where service provision and management structures are said to best reflect the needs of the community they serve.

In parallel with White Papers published for England, Scotland and Wales, 'Fit for the Future' (DHSS 1998) indicates the broad approach to the abolishment of the internal market and the GP fundholding scheme, through the promotion of partnership in the provision of health and personal social care in Northern Ireland.

Interpreted in strict terms, this would indeed reduce bureaucracy and drive down costs, because partnerships, being based upon trust, are much more easily administered. There is a problem however with the term 'partnership' and therefore with the cost of administration, for the very simple reason that one partner in a firm or organisation, or marriage, does not *commission* another partner to provide.

What the government appears to have in mind is more akin to strategic alliances, which increasingly are being used in the commercial world (e.g. big supermarket chains). These are devices which forge much closer links in the supply chain between the supplier, the distributing organisation and the customer.

However, 'Fit for the Future' claims that the government believes that in England the proposed changes will save billions of pounds and, scaled down to Northern Ireland size, this can be translated into a saving of £25 million. It seems that the only way to achieve this target might be to reduce the way the current structure is administered and comments were invited from interested parties on two particular models:

- **Model A** Boards would concentrate on a more strategic role. Local commissioning would be carried out by primary care groups serving populations of 60 000–100 000.
- **Model B** Six to eight local care agencies with populations of between 200 000 and 300 000 replace existing Boards and some Trusts. Primary Care Partnerships with populations of between 25 000 and 50 000 would commission most services.

In the light of problems created by the disparate nature of internal approaches together with other ethical

Managing health and social services in Northern Ireland

considerations, the government is keen to see that there is a coordinating influence upon quality management for both health and social care. Part of its promotion will become key elements of future business planning. Initiatives include:

- the introduction of nationwide evidence-based frameworks to ensure consistent access to quality services;
- creation of a National Institute for Clinical Excellence (NICE) that will:
  — provide a lead in clinical and cost effectiveness,
  — draw up guidelines, and
  — ensure adequate dispersal throughout the country;
- creation of a Commission for Health Improvement (CHI) that will:
  — support and oversee quality in clinical services,
  — tackle shortcomings, and
  — engage in necessary intervention;
- imposition of a duty upon providers to ensure quality of care through sound clinical governance;
- provision of clear incentives for improvement in performance and sanctions where there are perceived deficiencies;
- regulation of the social care workforce and training through a General Social Care Council, which will also include arrangements for the development and maintenance of competencies; and
- registration and inspection arrangements for day and domicilliary care.

The situation in Northern Ireland is characterised by continuous change, and thus core principles may be applied in different ways. What is clear, however, is that the people of Northern Ireland are committed to achieving a good quality of service from the resources they have available to them, and that those who have charge of these resources, as in other parts of the UK, take the task most seriously.

References

DHSS (1998) Fit for the future. A consultation document on the government's proposals for the future of the Health and Personal Social Services in Northern Ireland. Belfast: DHSS.

Department of Health, Social Services and Public Safety (1999) Executive Information Service, 29 November.

Application 2:3 *Marion Andrews-Evans*

The new NHS in Wales

In this application, Marion Evans outlines key points related to the provision of health care in Wales which have emerged as part of the UK devolution agenda.

As in all other countries in the UK, during 1998 and 1999 the health service in Wales underwent considerable changes. In fact it was the first time in the history of the NHS that every level of the service was affected by organisational change, from the health department at the Welsh Office, through Trusts and Health Authorities, right down to the general practices.

THE NATIONAL ASSEMBLY FOR WALES

On 1 July 1999 the National Assembly for Wales was established. Although it has no primary legislative powers, it does have devolved responsibility for the delegation of its budgets between the public services in Wales, including the health service. The Assembly has to operate within the legislation of the 1999 Act as established by Westminster, but it does have the power to allocate resources to the health service and make decisions on how the Act is enacted in Wales. Because of these powers, the NHS in Wales is different in many respects from the NHS in other UK countries, and the Act is implemented to meet the local needs of the Welsh people and the health professionals working in the Principality.

The National Assembly is organised into secretariats, with NHS Wales coming under the secretary for health and social services. Within the Assembly is the Health

Department, which has been organised along similar lines to the English NHS Executive, with a director of NHS Wales and a management board which includes the medical and nursing directors as well as directors for human resources, strategy and performance.

NHS TRUSTS

During 1998 a decision was made to merge all Trusts in Wales, and from 1 April to establish 16 new Trusts, considerably larger than the previous organisations, with the majority of Trusts being integrated acute, community and mental health services. These changes were considered to be beneficial for patients as they would encourage better continuity of care and promote opportunities for multidisciplinary professional and service development. It would also ensure organisational stability for Trusts should Primary Care Trusts (or their Welsh equivalent) be established.

Of course, organisations with turnovers of over £250 million and employing up to 10 000 staff offer their own challenges, and new styles of devolved management have to be developed to ensure that the benefits are achieved and organisational risks are managed.

HEALTH AUTHORITIES

There are five Health Authorities in Wales, which were formed following mergers between Family Health Services Authorities and Health Authorities in 1996. Because of the considerable reduction in Health Authority numbers at that time it was agreed that the number of Health Authorities should not be reduced further. Their influence was strengthened in the areas of planning. They have responsibility for producing the Health Improvement Programmes (HImPs) and also for the management of performance.

In Wales there are no regional offices, thus Health Authorities are directly accountable to the Health Department of the National Assembly. In addition, roles undertaken by regions are split between the Health Authorities and the Health Department. The main result of this for Health Authorities is that they are much closer to

The broad context of health care

central decision making, but are also more influenced by political processes and the individual Assembly members. Because of the opportunity for personal contact with Assembly members and senior staff in the Health Department, the Health Authorities are able to have direct involvement in the development of NHS policy.

In consideration of the fact that it is not feasible for individual Health Authorities to commission certain high cost, low volume specialties, the Welsh Assembly has established the Specialist Health Service Commission for Wales.

LOCAL HEALTH GROUPS

Twenty-two Local Health Groups (LHGs) were established from 1 April 1999 as subcommittees of the Health Authorities. All LHGs are coterminous with the 22 local authorities, to promote and encourage inter-agency working and service planning.

The direction for their establishment came in the White Paper issued by the Welsh Office in January 1998 entitled 'NHS Wales: Putting Patients First' (Welsh Office 1998a) and expanded in the consultation paper 'Establishing Local Health Groups' (Welsh Office 1998b). To date, the Welsh Assembly has not agreed for LHGs in Wales to become Trusts, nor indicated the expected direction of LHGs at present.

As fundholding is no longer active in the NHS, LHGs have taken on the role of developing long-term agreements (LTAs) with Trusts, with the aim of involving local GPs in this new commissioning process. The main responsibilities of LHGs are listed in Box 2.3.1.

Box 2.3.1 Main responsibilities of the Welsh Local Health Groups

- To identify local need and draw up local health action plans (LHAPs) to improve health and health services, and to contribute to the Health Authority's HIP.
- To develop and improve primary care services and work to integrate these with community care in local settings.
- To determine what local services should be commissioned by involving other partners, e.g. local authorities and voluntary organisations in the process.
- To involve, consult and respond to the local community.

The new NHS in Wales

To carry out the responsibilities listed in Box 2.3.1 the LHGs will be managed by a governing body. Up to 18 members are permitted on the LHG Board, and there is wider representation than in PCGs.

The membership of the Board consists of:

6 general practitioners
2 nurses, midwives or health visitors (one to be a practice nurse)
2 Health Authority representatives
2 local authority representatives (one to be the director of social services)
1 optometrist
1 dentist
1 pharmacist
1 voluntary sector representative
1 lay member from the local community
the general manager of the LHG.

This is a large Board, and its ability to undertake specific areas of work and to make decisions could be challenged. To overcome this, subgroups of the LHG have been developed. These vary in structure in different LHGs, but all are required to have a clinical governance group, with a Board member taking lead responsibility for clinical governance. Commonly the lead is a local GP, but any health professional on the Board might undertake the role, so in some cases nurses fulfil these positions. The guidance for clinical governance activity and improving the quality of health services is contained in the Welsh Office document 'Quality Care and Clinical Excellence' (Welsh Office 1998c). A typical subgroup arrangement for a Local Health Group management is shown in Figure 2.3.1.

All LHG Boards have an appointed chairman. The local GPs on the Board have the first opportunity to demonstrate an interest in this role, if none is interested then another Board member will be elected. The day-to-day management of the LHG is overseen by an executive committee, which consists of some members of the Board including the chairman and general manager. The general manager (chief executive equivalent in PCGs) is the most senior member of the staff in the LHG and is accountable for its management. This appointment is made by the Health Authority, rather than the LHG Board.

An interesting dimension of the LHG management team is that local authority officers serve on the LHG Board. This

The broad context of health care

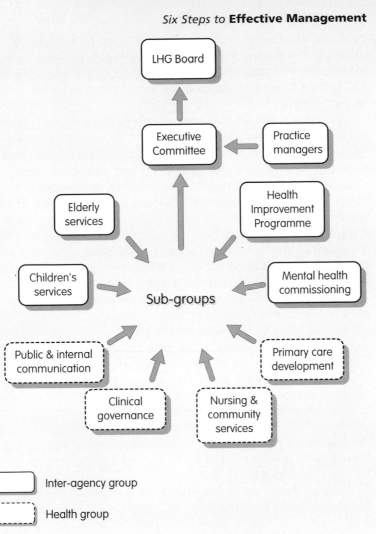

Figure 2.3.1 Typical stucture of a Local Health Group management subgroup.

aims to ensure and demonstrate commitment to the spirit of partnership working outlined in the White Paper, by action at a local level.

PARTNERSHIPS

The Welsh Office produced a guidance document entitled 'Partnership for Improvement' (Welsh Office 1998d). It included clear directions on how the new powers under the Health Act could provide opportunities for joint working

The new NHS in Wales

between local authorities and health services in Wales. As illustrated in Figure 2.3.1, there are many opportunities for inter-agency relationships within LHGs; often a group will be chaired by an individual from a non-health service department.

At present, the key focus of partnership working is joint planning and commissioning activity. This works to ensure a better coordinated provision of service, to better meet the needs of local people and also to achieve maximum cost-effectiveness. The strongest links are between health and social services, and these are reflected in the structure at the National Assembly, which supports the joint secretary post.

But partnerships are not only with statutory bodies. The inclusion of the voluntary sector as well as service users and carers is of equal importance in Wales today if services are really going to change. The ability to pool budgets and identify lead commissioners will also break down barriers that prevent continuity of service provision.

An excellent example of inter-agency working is the development of a joint mental health strategy. Together, the health and the social services, along with service users and voluntary bodies, identified service gaps, taking into account the needs of the clients. From this a joint local plan was developed that has resulted in jointly funded service developments, that really make a difference to local people. An example of this is a home respite service for the elderly mentally ill, jointly funded by health and social services and run by the voluntary sector.

Further developments will include the possibility of building shared facilities such as integrated day hospitals and centres, as well as provide bed facilities to use flexibly between health and social care.

Partnership working is clearly the way ahead. However, in all the enthusiasm for 'joined-up' working, managers must not lose sight of their core business, and must ensure that they continue to meet the health needs of their population.

BETTER HEALTH – BETTER WALES

A strategic framework entitled 'Better Health – Better Wales' was issued in October 1998 (Welsh Office 1998e). This document specifically gave direction to the Welsh NHS and its partners on promoting good health in the population. Though much of the White Paper 'NHS Wales: Putting Patients First' focuses on the treatment and care of the sick, it also emphasises the importance of improving health and wellbeing in the population by the prevention of disease. Still working within the partnership model, 'Better Health – Better Wales' identifies a framework through which the population's health can be improved. The framework names four key areas: alliances, communities, children, and environment and lifestyle.

Within this strategy, the development of local health alliances (National Assembly for Wales 1999) is seen as crucial. These alliances are led by the local authority and each LHG area will have an alliance which will contribute a public health and health promotion dimension. Each alliance will represent local interests from local councillors, voluntary and private care sectors, police, probation, local authority departments as well as local businesses. The key work of the alliance is to assess local health status and contributory factors, and then together identify areas for target action, e.g. to reduce road accidents in children. These alliances currently are in their infancy, but their focus on local action has the potential for making a real difference to health.

HEALTH SERVICE VALUES

To be a manager in the NHS can be stressful, particularly at a time of such significant change. As part of the change processes the National Assembly has provided direction for the health service and its staff by outlining how the service should be managed and delivered. Eight service values have been identified to inform the work, planning and delivery of services in the NHS throughout Wales (Box 2.3.2).

> **Box 2.3.2**
>
> - Fairness
> - Effectiveness
> - Integration
> - Accountability
> - Efficiency
> - Flexibility
> - Responsiveness
> - Promoting independence

The new NHS in Wales

Six Steps to **Effective Management**

References

National Assembly for Wales (1999) Developing local health alliances. Cardiff: Welsh Office.

Welsh Office (1998a) NHS Wales: putting patients first. London: The Stationery Office

Welsh Office (1998b) Establishing local health groups. Cardiff: Welsh Office.

Welsh Office (1998c) Quality care and clinical excellence. Cardiff: Welsh Office.

Welsh Office (1998d) Partnership for improvement. Cardiff: Welsh Office.

Welsh Office (1998e) Better health – better Wales – a strategic framework. Cardiff: Welsh Office.

Chapter **Three**

Quality in health – new agendas

Brian Edwards

- • **Some parameters**
- • **A first class service**
- • **Variation in quality**

- • **National standards**
- • **Performance monitoring**
- • **References**

OVERVIEW

Quality always has been high on the agenda of those providing health care in both the NHS and the private sector, but never more integrated into the whole business of health care than it is today. In this chapter, Brian Edwards takes us through the key issues, and points out the links between centre policy and care delivery.

Quality in health care is challenging territory. How is it to be defined and who is to judge? A professional judgement may not coincide with that of the patient, whose frame of reference may be very different. Every time the public is asked how the NHS might be improved they place reductions in waiting lists close to the top of the list. Many professionals, however, regard short waiting lists as not only impracticable but also a gross distortion of their clinical priorities. Patients value convenience and timeliness but the system is organised to value more highly the time of the health professional. Patients value communication skills very highly indeed, but this skill is not one that is seriously tested in professional training.

Even in territory such as drug trials, and the economic evaluation of new compounds, one finds sharp conflicts. A new cancer drug may not increase life span at all and thereby fail the economic hurdle for use in the NHS. The fact that it sharply reduces nausea is not valued highly enough to tip the scales. Interestingly, it is widely prescribed in private practice. Some would judge that much of the surgery undertaken on patients within months of death from diseases like cancer produces no real benefit but much discomfort. In this sense at least, quality questions assume an ethical dimension.

SOME PARAMETERS

Those who lead the NHS talk about it as being amongst the best in the world. The public appears to agree … or do they? Could it be that consistently high ratings are not for the service the NHS provides at a patient level but for the value of living in a society where health care is free at the point of need? Until recently, measures of the quality of the patient's experience and the outcome of treatment were poor. The temperature of the food was measured and commented upon more often than the treatment the patient received. How many months patients waited for surgery was recorded, but little was known about what happened when they were treated. 'Did the treatment work?' was a question rarely asked with any force outside the immediate clinical team. The huge investment made in clinical audit during the Thatcher years developed as a weak educational tool for those professionals who were interested. It hardly touched the poor performers who had most to learn from the results. The NHS has always had plenty of professionals and managers trying very hard to measure and improve the quality of health care on their patch or in their specialty. Often it worked, but it was usually transitory because it was dependent upon them. When they moved on or circumstances changed standards slipped back.

The system had no means of locking the improvements into practice so that they could weather the turbulence of high rates of staff change and movement. Over many years, the culmination of all this effort has had an impact, and standards have gradually improved. The NHS is undoubtedly better in terms of clinical quality than it was 20 years ago. But it is a very slow

The broad context of health care

process and huge variations are still apparent throughout the system.

A FIRST CLASS SERVICE

The search for a national quality strategy took a number of years and a number of false starts. It took a new government to break through and this they did, at least at a conceptual level in 1998, when Frank Dobson, the then secretary of state for health, launched 'A First Class Service: Quality in the New NHS' (Department of Health 1998a). The key elements of this strategy for England are given in Box 3.1.

These principles were reinforced by a new statutory duty of quality, which was incorporated in the 1999 Health Act as follows: 'It shall be the duty of Health Boards, Special Health Boards and NHS Trusts to put and keep in place arrangements for the purpose of monitoring and improving the quality of health care which it provides to individuals.' It will be fascinating to see how the courts interpret this when the challenge comes … as it will.

> **Box 3.1** Key elements of 'A First Class Service: Quality in the New NHS'
>
> - Everybody should get high quality care. Unacceptable variations should end.
> - Clinical decisions should be based on the best possible evidence of effectiveness.
> - Treatment should be delivered with courtesy and a real understanding of patients' fears and worries.
> - High quality and cost effectiveness are two sides of the same coin.
> - A new National Institute for Clinical Excellence (NICE) should ensure authoritative national guidance is available on the latest drugs and technologies.
> - National Service Frameworks (NSFs) should lay down the care that patients should expect.
> - Clinical governance policies should ensure that such standards are met locally.
> - A Commission for Health Improvement (CHI) should check that standards are being met.
> - A new national survey of patient and user experience should be carried out.
> - High standards of professional regulation are necessary.

Quality in health – new agendas

VARIATION IN QUALITY

Some degree of variation in quality is inevitable, particularly if there is evidence of continuous improvement. As prime minister, Margaret Thatcher had spotted variations in efficiency (for example in the lengths of hospital stay) which she thought would be levelled out by competition. She was partly right but enormous variations remained, as the performance tables produced by the Department of Health in November 1998 demonstrate (Table 3.1).

At that time Frank Dobson, secretary of state for health, also spotted variations in treatment. For example, in one region, amongst 35 surgeons, rates of mastectomy for breast cancer varied from nil (meaning that all women had breast conservation surgery) to 80%. Knee replacement surgery is highly effective in removing pain yet the range of access across the country is between 18 and 62 per 100 000 population. Fertility treatment is available in some parts of the country but not in others.

The first stage in dealing with variations is to measure them and this is why league tables are so popular, and, it must be said, so effective. People do react to pictures of their relative performance once they have been through the stage of arguing about the numbers being incorrect. Building performance mirrors is a key part of the task of any management team. Often just building an accurate mirror is enough to stimulate and sustain quality. The best organisations have real time mirrors.

The range of variation also represents an enormous opportunity for improvement by rolling up the bottom half of poor performance. If the patients who found themselves in the lower quartile of cancer care could receive a higher standard, the

Table 3.1 Examples from Department of Health NHS performance tables 1998

Operation	Low £	High £	Average £
Cataract	337	1659	699
Hip replacement	1834	6494	3678
Vasectomy	148	1000	332
Appendectomy	468	2108	1114

From Department of Health (1998b)

The broad context of health care

result would be dramatic. The barrier is not usually cash, but the quality of clinical organisation.

NATIONAL STANDARDS

In a service that is national, some overall standard setting is necessary and this is what the new National Service Frameworks are designed to secure. To begin with the Frameworks will be specialty based, but over time they will become industry wide and no doubt encompass the independent and private sectors. Greg Dyke, in his recent review of the Patient's Charter, has also recommended a small range of minimum national standards, although he ended up recommending local charters rather than a national one (Department of Health 1998c). To be really powerful, such standards have to be strictly enforced and, once consolidated, moved on. But in modern Britain one always has to remember that devolution in Scotland, Wales and Northern Ireland will accentuate variation. These factors are addressed in more detail in Chapter 2.

The new National Service Frameworks will build on the earlier work on cancer which was more concerned with the organisation of services than with the actual treatment protocols. This emphasis on organisation will be very distinctive in the early models as they deal with, for example, which services are best provided in primary care, in general hospitals and specialist centres. Mental health and coronary heart disease are the first subject areas.

NICE, the special health authority that will produce the frameworks, started its work in 1999 and will also produce guidance for clinicians about effective treatments and the value and effectiveness of new drugs and medical devices. For the first time in the NHS there will be a single national focus for the work on clinical effectiveness. NICE is potentially a very important body indeed, with the power to influence profoundly clinical practice decisively. In its early years it will not find it difficult to find treatments that definitely do not work and others that definitely do. Eventually though, it will hit those treatments that work for some patients and not for others and where clinical opinion is sharply divided. Much medicine is not set in stone and the best results are only obtained when evidence is applied together with clinical instinct and experience. Even the human genome, with its direct links between inherited genes and disease, is complicated by lifestyle and environment.

Quality in health – new agendas

81

PERFORMANCE MONITORING

'How are we doing?' is a question that is second nature to successful organisations. It reflects a passionate desire to keep up standards, to know when standards have dropped and to keep up with the competition. It is done best in real time with constant quality checks and challenges when standards approach danger point. Many of these checks are automatic (like temperature controls) but others are built into staff training and organisational culture. In these organisations quality becomes both an obsession and a routine.

Getting a public sector organisation to perform to such standards represents an enormous challenge. The performance review mechanisms are almost always historical and conducted from above. The question is 'how did they do?' rather than 'how did we do?'. To make matters worse, the patients or clients have only a limited range of alternatives and professional attitudes are shaped by the service rationing they are expected to undertake as they decide who is most deserving of their skills.

Rationing is a fertile breeding ground for professional arrogance and self-importance. The way through these problems for the NHS is the development of what is termed 'clinical governance'. This is the elixir that will 'create an environment in which excellence in clinical care will flourish'. It is, on the one hand, a clear set of corporate values and rules and on the other, a set of commitments about investment in professional staff. It also represents a commitment to measure and evaluate clinical care with a rigor that has been noticeably absent in the past. Making the chief executives of the NHS Trusts carry ultimate responsibility for assuring quality is tough but appropriate. It leaves unanswered the question as to the accountability of professional heads who always saw themselves as being responsible for professional standards. This opens up the possibility of a chief executive interfering directly in what was previously regarded as private professional territory.

Clinical audit programmes produce historical data on some aspects of clinical performance but were built on the foundations of professional education and to many have been a great disappointment. For the most part they still only capture segments of the patient's total experience anyway, as few have managed to connect the audit processes in hospital to those in primary care. In the new world of the NHS these processes will be strengthened. The big four national confidential inquiries into preoperative deaths, still births and infant deaths, maternal deaths and suicides and homicides by people with mental illness will come under the umbrella of NICE. This will, it is thought, give greater clarity and coherence to the status of their findings. All relevant hospital doctors and other health professionals will be required to participate. But why are these inquiries conducted in private and with a high degree of anonymity for the professionals concerned? The answers lie in deeply entrenched attitudes to clinical freedom and a fear that if anonymity is not promised nobody will participate for fear of the consequences (including civil proceedings by patients for damages).

The teeth of the new drive for quality in the NHS is going to be in the Commission for Health Improvement. This organisation will carry out local reviews of performance as well as conducting the national survey of patient and user experience. This is more than the Health Advisory Service writ large, for it will have substantial powers of intervention as well. Maintaining a balance between the need for consistent high quality and legitimate clinical freedom is going to be testing.

But when the Commission fails to resolve an issue, governments will still, no doubt, resort to even more expensive solutions, such as judicial inquiries. The recent independent inquiry into Ashworth Special Hospital cost £2.5 million (Department of Health 1999). The Bristol Inquiry will cost substantially more. Such inquiries, with their heavy legal component, have to be reserved for only those circumstances where the events are extremely serious and the public need reassuring that any inquiry really is independent. The legal process, with its formality and attention to details, is indeed a powerful audit tool when in inquisitorial mode.

The outstanding challenge for all health systems is to make them work reliably and consistently. As they become more complicated and ever more reliant on the skills of specialists from different disciplines they struggle to cope and suffer from regular and persistent system failure. The patient does not receive the appropriate treatment, not because it is judged to be ineffective or too expensive, but because the system fails to deliver it. Thirty years ago medical science discovered how to prevent antibodies from rhesus negative women attacking the fetus. A simple injection of anti-D does the trick perfectly. However, 50 babies a year still slip though the net. Their mothers never got their anti-D.

Thousands of men and women die each year from heart attacks which might have been treatable had they received a

Quality in health – new agendas

thrombolytic within 90 minutes. Some of these people lived in remote rural areas but the majority lived in the cities. They might have been saved if the system had worked for them. The guidance on the administration of anticoagulants prior to surgery is clear. Many patients do not receive it. Many of the patients in the special hospitals should not be there. Their admission was the consequence of a lottery. They could have ended up in prison just as easily.

The problems of coordination now stretch well beyond the boundaries of individual hospitals or clinical teams. In the treatment of cancer a patient's pathway will usually involve at least two hospitals and their primary care team. One response to this is to create clinical networks that knit everything together for individual patients. In Northern Ireland they are planning to create one single integrated clinical network for serious illness and emergencies (Northern Ireland Office 1998). Thus the local accident service run by skilled nurses will be an integral part of the emergency network. Links by modern technologies will allow immediate consultation and professional support.

Often, the consequences of system failure is simply delay or inconvenience but sometimes it can be far more serious. The hunt is on for those parts of the clinical process where the consequences of failure are so dangerous that this particular bit must be made fault free. It is possible to make some features of a clinical process guaranteed fault free. It requires a strong professional consensus about what is right, strict professional discipline and routine and automatic control and alert systems. At one extreme might be the automatic calibration of radiotherapy machines to ensure patients are actually receiving the prescribed dose. At the other might be a process that ensured that no patient could enter the operating theatre until their anticoagulant status had been confirmed. The compulsory preflight checklists undertaken by pilots could equally be applied to surgery, and not just for some surgeons or some of the time but for all surgeons all of the time. Routine and repetition are often at the heart of high-quality processes.

The greatest assurance of quality in health care lies in the attitude and skills of the staff involved. Recent years have seen moves to enforce continuing professional development and this seems highly appropriate in a fast moving world where keeping up-to-date is a real challenge. The time for automatic relicensing at regular intervals is not far away.

But the debate about the future is far from over. The tension between national standards and local priorities will remain. The

The broad context of health care

extent to which the clinical freedom of individual professionals can be circumscribed by protocol is a challenging question. We know that quality by inspiration is transitory unless any gains are locked into routine professional processes. We know that quality is also a product of a long-term and substantial investment in the skills and attitudes of staff – all staff, not just professional staff. Quality is not produced as a result of a 10-year plan. Real quality is deeply engrained in the culture of organisations and businesses. It is second nature and engineered in to be routine and expected. It can survive changes in leadership.

References

Department of Health (1998a) A first class service. Quality in the new NHS. London: The Stationery Office.

Department of Health (1998b) National schedule of reference costs. London: The Stationery Office.

Department of Health (1998c) Report on the new NHS charter. London: The Stationery Office.

Department of Health (1999) Report of the Committee of Inquiry into the Personality Disorder Unit at Ashworth Special Hospital. Vol 1. Cm 4194–11. London: The Stationery Office.

Northern Ireland Office (1998) Putting it right. The case for change in Northern Ireland's Hospital Service. Belfast: Northern Ireland Office.

Quality in health – new agendas

Application 3:1 *Peter Westhead*

Forget-me-not: a vision of care excellence

Peter Westhead has prepared a summary of the key factors within this important report (Audit Commission 2000) which addressed services in the public sector for older people with mental health problems. There is a number of important issues contained here. First, that of quality. In order that a quality service can be provided, it is important to see what is available, and if that fits the needs of the service users. Secondly, it makes the point, which is embedded in the notion of clinical governance, that partnerships are beneficial in providing excellent care. Care should be focused on the client, rather than being contained within professional and organisational parameters. Linked to this, the third point made is that, even with commitment to both quality and joint, collaborative working, if resources do not follow the client, out from hospital into the community, all efforts will be compromised.

Reports such as this one have a strategic role in shaping policy. Individual practitioners as well as organisations can utilise the findings to enhance their clients' experiences.

In the final 18 months of the twentieth century, the Audit Commission undertook a review of services provided by the public sector for older people with mental health problems. This led to the publication of a national report entitled 'Forget Me Not – Mental Health Services for Older People' (Audit Commission 2000). The theme of that report and those that follow from it is one of promoting independence for this group of people.

The report addresses the issues in the context of population trends and the health consequences of:

- more people living to an older age,
- more people with mental health problems,
- a quarter of those over 85 developing dementia,
- a third of those people needing constant supervision,
- 10–16% over 65 developing clinical depression, and
- people with severe and enduring mental health problems, such as schizophrenia, also growing older.

Family carers often are under great stress and knowing how to get help enables many to carry on caring. However, the report suggests that approximately half of carers did not have the problem explained to them, nor were they informed of what to expect in the future. Less than one half of GPs felt that they had received sufficient training to diagnose and manage dementia.

The cost of caring has been estimated at over £6 billion per annum. The government sees mental health for older people as a priority and commissioning groups are being required to develop integrated plans and identify gaps in services, and to facilitate arrangements such as the pooling of resources to allow closer working partnerships between health services and social services to emerge. New standards are to be published to provide a National Service Framework (NSF) for services for older people. Primary Care Groups (PCGs) will focus these services by aiming to provide:

- early help
- specialised home-based services
- coordinated professional input and joint working of agencies
- comprehensive, shared strategies
- audited progress.

The Audit Commission report surveyed 12 geographical areas, and obtained information from carers, general practitioners, specialist mental health services and other care agencies. Innovation and joint working had led to examples of flexible and responsive care. However, in asking questions of these groups it found, amongst other things, that:

Forget-me-not: a vision of care excellence

- only half of the carers surveyed said they had been told what help was available,
- many GPs felt ill-prepared to deal with mental health problems, fewer than half feeling that their training was adequate, and
- support by local mental health professionals for GPs increased GPs' belief in the value of early diagnosis of dementia and depression.

Specialist assessment (usually by the Community Mental Health Care Trust (CMHT) teams) of clients at home is often better, more accurate and involves the opinions and needs of carers. In the Audit Commission's findings, these specialist assessments did not always happen. It found that those people at home with mental health problems would benefit from a range of specialist services in their own homes to support their continuing care needs, as well as requiring support in the form of day centres, outpatient departments, and the opportunity to access respite care.

Most expenditure on specialist mental health care occurs in hospital and residential care, despite the fact that most people would prefer to be supported in their own homes. The report urged that Health Authorities and Trusts should respond by reconsidering the balance towards care being delivered within the community setting, and thus, Health Authorities need to respond to this by reallocation of funds.

Specialist community-based care includes community psychiatric nurses (CPNs), home care workers, day care, voluntary organisations, respite care, residential and nursing homes. However, the Commission found that the mix and availability varied in the areas surveyed. Specialist home care workers, trained to be better able to cope with difficult or challenging behaviours, provide continuity of care and coordinate more effectively with mental health teams, were employed in only five of the 12 areas visited. In those five areas, GPs were more satisfied with the services provided. A review of the skill-mix of community-based services was recommended.

Interestingly, in four of the 12 groups, the average level of dependency of people with dementia was very high, equivalent to that in residential care, suggesting that people attending day centres are being helped to stay at home.

At present the type of care at day centres depends more on the values and experiences of those who manage the centre and the levels of special training rather than the needs of the particular group of clients who use it. Joint staff planning is called for, and the report recommended that the most appropriate mix of staff should be used to meet the users' needs.

Respite care was often requested by carers to help them to continue caring. The provision of this was found to be variable. Most respite was provided in residential and nursing homes. The report said that the authorities should ensure sufficient respite care, and include some provision for respite care in clients' own homes.

When people with dementia are no longer able to stay at home, hospital care may be required. The report noted that areas with highly developed community services admitted fewer people to hospital, and only then with the objective of treating severe symptoms or stabilising unmanageable behaviour, before discharging clients back to community care.

Effective communication between all members of the physical health services and mental health services is seen as essential by the Commission. Most users have complex needs. Residential or nursing care is sometimes required, but it is the most expensive option. The report recommended that the decision to take this option should always take into account the views of users/carers and of other professionals. Specialist homes for the elderly mentally ill exist, and a third of their admissions comes from other homes. This suggests that the needs of the clients could not be fully met in those environments. It was noted that better support within all the residential homes may avoid the need for clients to be moved and the report went on to advise that once admitted, progress reviews should occur at 3–6 month intervals and staff advised and supported, particularly where the home is not a specialised unit.

The quality of care provided by staff and the environment in which this care is delivered are crucial factors. Dementia care mapping was seen by the Commission as a significant factor in raising levels of knowledge and awareness among staff. Continuing care was not the policy in four of the Health Authorities surveyed. An interesting proposal is that staff might move between various care settings, rather than the resident moving around to go to the staff. This might provide

Forget-me-not: a vision of care excellence

flexible support across a range of care settings, and give staff a chance to practise in a number of contexts. The Health Act 1999 (Department of Health 1999) encourages health and social service organisations to pool funding, and this is likely to break down organisational barriers which have shaped care packages in the past.

Coordination and flexibility between services is seen as necessary in such complex service management. The care programme approach, originally proposed for younger people, could be adapted. Information sharing is seen as a crucial part of coordination of services, as is shared responsibility and flexibility. The most successful CMHT contained a mix of professionals working from the same office. The process of coordination needs to be managed by a key worker in order that best use can be made of all resources.

A comprehensive strategy to encompass Health Improvement Programmes (HImPs), joint commissioning and integrated staff policies should be developed. This might include the contribution of the voluntary organisations, the use of needs focused tactics and the effective management of quality information necessary to inform those strategies. When all groups of staff work together in the field, good practice can be more easily disseminated.

The report concludes with some key recommendations:

1. Primary care should provide competent support and advice.
2. Information should be easily accessible and available locally.
3. GPs require support from mental health specialists.
4. Assess clients at home where possible by members of a CMHT.
5. Resources should be balanced in favour of home-based services.
6. Specialist trained home care staff should be used.
7. Day provision should be specific and jointly provided by health and social services.
8. A range of respite options should include home and emergency services.
9. Hospital admissions are minimised by effective community support and close links with physical health care specialists.
10. Specialists should support nursing and residential homes.

11. NHS-funded continuing care should be determined jointly by health and social services.
12. Coordinated, integrated, flexible professionals will deliver the most effective care.
13. Care programme approach models of planning care or similar may be beneficial.
14. Shared information will facilitate more effective care.
15. Clear goals must be set balancing home care, day care, outpatients and hospital services.
16. Quality information is required to inform planning and monitoring quality.
17. Innovations, particularly where jointly commissioned, should be encouraged.

References

Audit Commission (2000) Forget me not – mental health services for older people. London: Audit Commission.
Department of Health (1999) The Health Act. London: Department of Health.

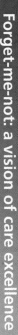

Forget-me-not: a vision of care excellence

Section **Two**

DELIVERING THE BUSINESS

OVERVIEW

From the big, strategic perspective of Section 1, we move on in Section 2 to the sharp end – the delivery of the business. More frequently now, those working in the health industry who are in the clinical professions are required to demonstrate management skills and knowledge in order that they can fulfil their roles; remember, quality now means not just giving the best service to the patient, but getting the best value for money from the resources available. The chapters in Section 2 will help you to do this. In Chapter 4, Linda Terry goes through the purposes and processes of business planning, and you see these techniques in action in different ways

Chapter 5 addresses the human resource elements, both in terms of the individual and the organisation, and the applications demonstrate this firstly in macrocosm, via the national workforce planning agenda, and then in the microcosm, as Jo Ouston points out that whilst it is important for each individual to have a development plan, these must be congruent with the bigger organisational picture.

In Chapter 6 Con Egan unravels the mysteries of financial activity in a most entertaining way, and Julie Gray demonstrates how she used some financial skills when she decided that she could better use resources at work. As a result of the changes Gray made, using financial acumen as well as her clinical judgement, the patients using the services of the assessment clinic receive a better quality of care.

Rose Stephens, Julia Bradbury and Richard Romaniak in Chapter 7 demonstrate how budgets are managed on a day-to-day basis, and Robert Dredge takes you through how to read a budget statement. Eva Lambert's Chapter 8 follows on from this, as she explains, and gives examples in the applications of the processes which lead to the delivery of cost-effective services.

To round this section off, Mike Cook in Chapter 9 looks at how effective management of the quality agenda gets translated into patient care. Julie Hyde goes on to demonstrate this, via a management example as she highlights the process of risk management, and sets it within the framework of clinical governance.

Delivering the business

Chapter **Four**

The contribution of business planning

Linda Terry

- **The purpose and benefits of planning**
- **Features of service and public sector organisations**
  The political agenda
  Performance issues for managers in planning and delivering services
- **The theory of planning**
  The strategic framework
  Operational planning
  The rational planning model
  Emergent planning
- **The planning framework: preparing a business case**
  Step one: the corporate mission
  Step two: scanning the external environment

- Step three: scanning the internal environment
  Step four: identifying opportunities and threats
  Step five: defining objectives
- **Structure of the plan**
  Rationale
  Objectives
  Operational planning
  Contingency planning
  Evaluation and control
- **Why plans fail**
- **Conclusion**
- **References**
- **Further Reading**

OVERVIEW

As the effective management of resources is an integral part of management, the ability to plan for activity, at either a macro level (e.g. whole Trust) or micro level (e.g. ward) becomes more important. This responsibility does not lie only with management. Every health professional has a role to play and a contribution to make. Collaboration and partnership are key values in the business planning process. The member of staff nearest to the service delivery is often in a position to make a crucial contribution to the planning cycle, as they are likely to know the details of that particular service, and thus where the sticking points might be. This 'grassroots' knowledge combined with a grasp of the big picture of health strategy is most likely to result in a flexible, workable plan.

The term 'business plan' is a generic one. In general usage it refers to the process outlined in this chapter. However, a business plan can focus on a particular service need.

The techniques of business planning can be used to inform large or small tasks, from implementing a new strategy to operationalising a new system. It may be that a whole new service is being contemplated, implying significant resource consequences and changes to established processes and practices, or alternatively, the introduction of new technology with similar demands on resources and staff development may be necessary. In either case, planning can help managers and staff to avoid potential pitfalls and achieve the desired outcomes effectively.

This chapter will consider the benefits of planning, examine several planning models and techniques and also look at some of the pitfalls, particularly where constant change is a feature of working life. And it will look at why plans fail.

THE PURPOSE AND BENEFITS OF PLANNING

'Why do we plan?' may seem to be an unnecessary question. The alternative might be to operate in the equivalent of a fog, without direction and subject to the impact of every external or internal change: an environment in which there is no control. A counterargument may be that planning is redundant in a health service that is subject to constant upheaval and where a 6-month plan can be regarded as long term. In this environment the new skills for managers, whether at strategic or operational level, may be less to do with the ability to forward plan than

> **Box 4.1** Attributes of planning at its best
>
> ● It is a structured means of analysing an issue or problem
> ● It evolves from a vision of progress or aim
> ● It involves staff in its development
> ● It confers ownership of goals
> ● It is an aid to communication
> ● It is a means of control in relation to the implementation of objectives

the ability to adapt, adjust services and operate perpetually in a short-term framework, whilst tolerating a high level of ambiguity.

Why plan if there is no control of resources, no certainty of continuity? This scenario is likely to be the environment with which most managers are familiar. But the argument is not for the abolition of planning but an acceptance of its conditional nature. An understanding of good planning and good management combined can limit the potential for confusion and dissatisfaction and provide a cohesive framework which coordinates the allocation of resources, channelling them towards the achievement of agreed goals.

The phrase 'agreed goals' highlights an essential point: if a manager undertakes planning in isolation, the plan will at worst fail and at best be only partially achieved. Failure to consult, failure to communicate, failure to involve staff in implementation equate to failure to succeed. According to Johns & Scholes (1997) planning at its best has the attributes listed in Box 4.1. It is clear that planning can become a way of working, not only for a manager but for the team. But the rider to that statement is that a rigid approach to planning can be just as much an impediment to success as a lack of a planning framework. Successive sections in the chapter will demonstrate the need for flexibility and adaptability within the planned framework.

FEATURES OF SERVICE AND PUBLIC SECTOR ORGANISATIONS

Features that distinguish the planning process within the public sector environment are the political agenda, the rise of consumerism and the presence of performance management when planning and delivering services.

The political agenda

Even within the relatively small environment of a hospital ward or GP practice planning cannot take place in isolation or without recognition of the national and local conditions in which the health service operates. The Thatcher era introduced the concept of the market and the principles of competition into the NHS in an effort to increase cost-effectiveness and greater efficiency through local accountability. Regardless of government initiatives in the late 1990s to dismantle the internal market, it is clear that some aspects of the previous strategy will continue to affect the delivery of services and, therefore, the way that managers manage. Competition may be replaced by collaboration, decentralisation may be replaced by increasing state direction and intervention, but the quasi-market and, in particular, the demarcation of services between the public and private sectors are unlikely to disappear. Brooks & Weatherston (1997, p. 279), rewriting Brown and Jackson's statement made in 1992 describing the dominance of the public sector in health service delivery, note the shift from public sector reliance to a mixed market as follows:

> Most of us born in the United Kingdom were born in quasi-independent NHS Trusts where many of our mothers rented a private room, were tended by GP fundholding doctors and paid full market rate prescription charges, were educated in private or grant-maintained schools and private or quasi-independent universities as no-grant, fee-paying 'customers' ... will be nursed in private nursing homes and will be cremated and buried on EU 'Set-Aside' farming land or other privatised graveyards by our dependants.

This gives a clear indication of the mixed public/private sector economy.

The trend to public/private market sector interdependence will be maintained partly because of the national strategic imperative to control costs through implicit, if no longer explicit, competition and through the inability of the public sector to provide all the services envisaged in the 1947 Act which created the NHS.

The introduction of the Patient's Charter in 1991 and the accompanying rise in customer/consumer expectations and associated demands for compensation as part of the Conservative government's competitive strategy have placed increased demands on the provision of health care. Demands for increased service delivery continue to impact on local managers working with diminishing resources.

The combined impact of these issues on local managers will continue to be experienced in the management of limited resources, a continuing focus on the value for money (VFM) factor and increasing demand for evidence of clinical effectiveness. Managers are required increasingly to demonstrate the evidence base for their planning decisions and operations, and both to be cost-effective and clinically effective.

Performance issues for managers in planning and delivering services

There are specific issues for managers working in service industries in controlling cost and quality. It is worth looking at what is meant by performance management when planning services. What is a service and what are some of its characteristic features? And why does understanding these concepts help with planning?

Kotler (1991, p. 455) defines a service as 'any activity or benefit that one party can offer another that is essentially intangible and does not result in the ownership of anything. Its production may or may not be tied to a physical product.' In health service terms, we can distinguish the application of a dressing (the service) from the dressing (the product) itself; or to give another example, from the making of an appointment from the appointment itself. In both cases, the delivery of the service is intrinsically linked to the person giving it. The issues relating to cost and control of the delivery of that service are subject, therefore, to the standard of performance from the member of staff giving that service. So how does this impact on the manager responsible for the planning and delivery of the service?

Cowell (1984) defines four qualities as distinguishing services from products (Box 4.2). He propounds that these distinguishing features create particular challenges for those responsible for the planning and delivery of services. For example, in the light of the variability of services, there are three issues for managers to consider: (a) the effective selection, recruitment and development of staff, (b) standardisation of the service-performance process and (c) customer satisfaction monitoring systems.

It is useful to recognise the centrality of these concepts in the business planning process – the impact of the external environment and the specific demands of service management and the interaction of the two. They will be referred to when we come to consider the planning framework.

> **Box 4.2**   Qualities that distinguish services from products
>
> *Intangibility*   A service cannot be seen, tasted or felt, for example, before it is used. Users base their assessment of the service on intangibles such as personal recommendation, past experience, image – they will draw inferences from the quality of the service from the people delivering it, the place, the price, the environment in which it is experienced.
>
> *Inseparability*   The person giving a service (i.e. dressing, appointment, consultation) is the service. As the user or customer is usually present at the giving of the service, provider–customer interaction becomes a defining feature.
>
> *Variability*   Services are highly varied, depending on who provides them and when and where they are provided.
>
> *Perishability*   A service cannot be stored. The wrong intervention is a wasted intervention; a missed appointment is a cost; supply and demand need managing (e.g. the management of winter bed provision) to minimise waste.

THE THEORY OF PLANNING

The strategic framework

> There are three types of companies: those who make things happen; those who watch things happen; those who wonder what happened.   (Anonymous)

Planning is employed by organisations who make things happen, who use circumstances to shape their organisations and who are not merely reactive to external and internal circumstances. The term 'strategic planning' is normally associated with senior management activity – but what does it actually mean?

Brooks & Weatherston (1997) define strategic planning as the attempt to match organisational capability with environmental opportunities. By definition, therefore, strategic planning is externally focused, shaping direction by recognising and responding to national and local initiatives. It is an attempt to formulate the goals and objectives of the whole organisation within a contemporary and forward-looking environment. It usually operates within a 3–5 year time span. Strategic planning uses many of the techniques employed in business planning.

Strategic planning at its best sets the direction for the organisation as a whole, providing vision and leadership for the

Delivering the business

> **Box 4.3** Examples of issues relevant to health service managers
>
> - Health Authority priorities: local commissioning
> - National strategic aims, such as 'Our Healthier Nation', National Service Frameworks
> - National budget: financial allocation to health services
> - Change in local demographics, e.g. rise in elderly population, creation of a new housing estate
> - Changes in the legislative or professional framework, e.g. review of the Nurses, Health Visitors and Midwives Act, post-registration education and practice (PREP), etc.

smaller units within it. It provides a framework for unit managers to plan, ensuring best use of resources within the whole organisation and diminishing the likelihood of individuals going off in a direction contrary to the stated aims of the whole. It builds on the organisation's strengths and purposes, ensuring a viable match between the external issues (Box 4.3) and internal competencies.

It is very often through strategic planning at senior management level that a 'vision' or 'mission statement' arises. At their best, such statements describe where the entire organisation is heading ('its purpose') and define the kind of organisation it aims to be ('value statement'). By definition, they also define what the organisation does not do and therefore can act as a central control. (Black and Decker's original mission statement 'making holes' was a clear statement of what they were and were not in business for.) It can be argued that, particularly in a climate of uncertainty, the vision statement should be a constant focus for all managers: a generalised statement of intent which the organisation as a whole focuses on and by which it maintains its direction when individual objectives are changed by circumstances.

Where vision or mission statements fail and become objects of derision (assuming staff are aware of them in the first place) is where the stated objectives and values of the organisation are felt to contrast with the realities experienced by staff at operational level. 'Investing in our staff' can be hard to swallow when staff numbers are reduced, training opportunities become limited and resources feel stretched beyond the acceptable. In such cases, the organisation's mission statement can be regarded as pie-in-the-sky (at best) and derided as hypocrisy (at worst). Mission statements should carry health warnings! But as a framework for shaping an organisation they have their merits.

The contribution of business planning

Drucker (1990) summarises the purposes of mission statements as being 'to focus on what the institution really tries to do and then do it so that everybody in the organisation can say: This is my contribution to the goal.' (p. 4).

So, in summary, the importance of strategic planning is in setting the direction for the organisation as a whole, enabling individual units to develop their own plans within a given and agreed framework. Good planning at this level

- diminishes the risk of failure,
- diminishes the likelihood of fragmentation and promotes cohesion (a pulling together, not apart),
- promotes best use of resources by defining objectives, and
- creates and communicates the vision and values of the organisation.

Operational planning

So how does operational planning differ from and relate to strategic planning? The aims created through strategic planning are necessarily generalised, establishing goals for the organisation as a whole. Operational planning creates goals which are more specific, more focused on a particular unit or individual employees. Consider the example in Box 4.4. This example highlights not only the difference in specificity between strategic and operational aims but also the direct relationship between the two in terms of purpose. Assuming for a moment that the flow of information into an organisation is always downward, the implementation of strategic planning can be modelled as shown in Figure 4.1. In operational planning, policies and procedures are developed by managers to implement defined aims. They

---

Box 4.4 The difference and relation between a strategic aim and an operational objective

'Delivering health care for the people of Anyshire' (*strategic aim*)

becomes

'Providing psychiatric health care and support for the children, adolescents and their families of Anyshire' (*operational aim*)

and even more specifically

'Developing an outreach team delivering child and adolescent psychiatric care for Area A within Anyshire by June 2001 within a defined annual budget of £x' (*operational objective*).

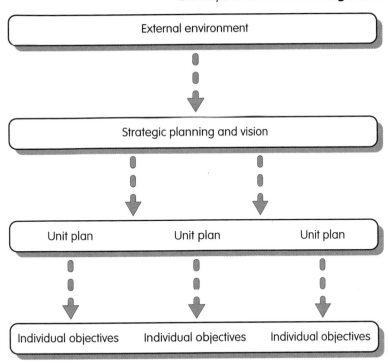

Figure 4.1 The implementation of strategic planning.

focus on tasks required of individual units or employees and lead to the identification of skills and resources to implement the objectives.

Operational planning can make use of techniques such as critical path analysis for the purposes of implementation and control. It is particularly useful for project management when a specific task has to be accomplished within a given time, budget and specification, as demonstrated in the example outlined in Box 4.5. Such plans are often seen visually expressed in Gantt charts where the graph expresses time on the horizontal axis and scheduled activities on the vertical axis. This visual representation allows managers to monitor the progress of the plan.

Clearly, planning with this degree of specificity enables progress to be audited and performance to be monitored. Control mechanisms can be inbuilt into operational planning at both unit and individual level. Management by objectives, individual performance review or appraisal and quality assessment indicators can be incorporated by managers to ensure that plans are not only implemented but evaluated and adapted according to the results.

The contribution of business planning

Box 4.5   Project management: an example

Objective
To introduce and evaluate a software package to monitor referrals within the unit within six months of start date and with a budget of £x.

Action plan
1. Identify information requirements in relation to the monitoring of referrals
2. Obtain technical advice in identifying appropriate software package
3. Identify staff training requirements
4. Identify pilot project to test system
5. Order software
6. Staff briefing
7. Identify staff training programme
8. Install software
9. Implement staff training programme
10. Commence pilot project
11. Pilot evaluation
12. Prepare contingency plan as result of evaluation
13. Implementation of full system for all referrals
14. Financial report against budget
15. Full evaluation
16. Define further action required (e.g. financial, technical, performance, information systems) as a result of evaluation

Timescale for action plan

Month 1	Month 2	Month 3	Month 4	Month 5	Month 6	Month 9
1,2,3,4,5	6,7	8,9	10	11,12	13,14	15,16

The rational planning model

The logical approach demonstrated in relation to operational planning leads us now to consider the place of the rational planning model in health care. Rational planning can be defined as 'a cycle of decisions which need to be made so that an organisation can achieve its objectives' (Lawton & Rose 1994, p. 125). It assumes a logical and linear progression of action resulting from the definition of solutions, controlled by the decision maker and implemented by identified units/individuals. Inherent in the model is the assumption of control over the environment and the organisation and hence it is associated with top-down management. Steps in the rational planning model are identified in Box 4.6.

According to the rational model, implementation of the plan requires:

- identification of resources to support the selected option,
- creation of control systems to monitor performance and provide information for evaluation, and

> **Box 4.6** Steps in rational planning
>
> Problem → Definition of the problem → Definition of the criteria for decisions → Identification of possible solutions and actions → Option appraisal → Selection of viable option → Implementation of solution → Feedback, evaluation and review.

- establishment of human resource systems and structures to facilitate implementation of the strategy (on the assumption that structure follows strategy).

Critically, the rational planning model assumes the following points are absolute:

- that there is a degree of certainty, viz. that the issue can be fully defined and that options can be clearly identified,
- that the environment (both external and internal) will not change,
- that the tasks have been properly identified,
- that decision makers are rational,
- that the required combination of resources is available,
- that those charged with implementation will carry out their task exactly as required,
- that clear communication between decision makers and those involved in implementation exists, and
- that no conflict of interest exists in the organisation.

Thus the rational planning model is best suited to an organisation which may be subject to limited change and which is operating in a stable environment. Even so, it may not produce the greatest benefits for the organisation, focusing as it does on control. Change management experience suggests that staff are better motivated to carry out tasks if they have been involved in the decision-making process, whereas this model assumes direction from the planners.

Emergent planning

An adaptation of the rational planning model is useful for organisations operating within unstable environments. This is emergent planning, where strategy 'evolves from activities taking place throughout the organisation and thus can be influenced by strategic planning via the rational model but is shaped by other influences as well' (Hatch 1997, p. 113). To operate in this framework an organisation sets broad aims and goals, providing guidance for managers but allowing individual units

The contribution of business planning

or managers to propose and implement policies and strategies of their own (Hatch 1997). The rationale for this model is that devolving responsibility to individuals is more likely to create responsiveness, adaptability and ownership than with an entirely directive approach. In this situation strategy can be influenced by structure as the parts inform the whole. Particular benefits of emergent strategic planning are that it provides:

- the opportunity for incremental planning to take place, i.e. small steps towards the achievement of the larger goal with the consequential reduction of risk of large-scale failure;
- the safety of agreeing small steps rather than aiming to achieve large goals in a climate of uncertainty;
- the opportunity for managers in differing units to negotiate and agree compromise/solutions around goals;
- the opportunity to develop creative solutions through enhanced participation;
- opportunism: the ability to exploit opportunities as they arise, unconstrained by the limits of a rigid corporate strategy; and
- the facility to test and adapt the plan against external signs.

This approach to planning has particular relevance in the health care sector. Health care organisations are usually characterised by clarity of general purpose, complexity of structure and a climate of change. In such situations it is unlikely that managers will be able to comprehend all aspects of the situation they are addressing, a situation which contradicts some of the basis assumptions for use of the rational planning model. Participation in planning by those charged with implementation (as in middle or unit managers) will create a more realistic and effective process wherein strategy will evolve from the existing systems and structures. The risks in such an approach are best summarised as fragmentation: the lack of a cohesive approach to a situation leading to missed opportunities and adverse effects on other sectors of the organisation if these are not considered.

THE PLANNING FRAMEWORK: PREPARING A BUSINESS CASE

Having looked at some of the issues surrounding planning, how do we go about developing a business case? Kotler's (1991) model of the strategic planning process (Fig. 4.2) provides a useful framework.

Delivering the business

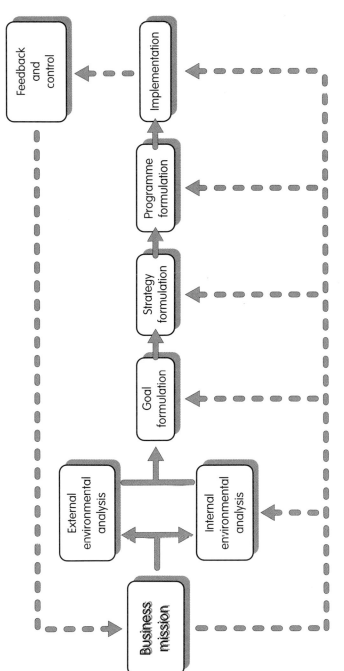

Figure 4.2 Framework for the strategic planning process.

The contribution of business planning

How does a middle or unit manager apply this when planning? Their particular aim might be to open a new unit or health centre, to introduce a new service or to consider extending a nursing home. What are the steps to take?

Step one: the corporate mission

We have stated earlier that the mission should define the aims and values of the whole organisation. So the first question to ask is: Does this aim fit in with the direction of the whole organisation? Is it likely to win the support of senior managers/partners/owners? If not, does it need rethinking and adapting or is it pointless to proceed? If the aim does fit with the general trend within the organisation, the manager can proceed to implement the next steps in the planning process.

Step two: scanning the external environment

The usual tool for scanning the external environment is the carrying out of a PEST (Political, Economic, Sociological, Technological) analysis (also known as a STEP analysis). Following these broad categories the manager can look at the external factors affecting his or her environment and assess their relevance to the particular goal being considered. Issues to consider could include the following.

Political
- Are there any government initiatives to hinder or advance the goal? (Are any hospital mergers planned or are there any care-in-the-community implications, for example?)
- Are there any local initiatives which could similarly influence the outcome? (e.g. health authority restraint on developments, where issues of internal competition or politics, (e.g. between management units) could influence the outcome of the plan).

Economic
- What budgetary or funding issues at national, local or organisational level might exert influence (i.e. hinder or advance) the aim?

Sociological

- Demographic trends: is the elderly population estimated to increase or decrease in your area?
- What might the impact of a new housing development locally be?
- Is the goal in line with cultural expectations (e.g. extension of services into the community, 'Health of the Nation' targets, consumer expectations)?
- Are there issues relating to the needs of the ethnic community to consider?

Technological

- What is happening in the world of technology which could affect the implementation of the goal?

Step three: scanning the internal environment

Having defined the external issues which might impact on the goal, the manager can proceed to a consideration of the internal environment. The SWOT (Strengths, Weaknesses, Opportunities, Threats) analysis is the tool usually adopted for this purpose. The organisation is examined in its totality: people, facilities, finances, estates, infrastructure and systems. What are the strengths of the organisation in relation to these functions? What are its weaknesses? And what effect will these have on the outcome of the goal in question? If the goal in question was, for example, the introduction of a new system of audit, the SWOT audit could reveal:

> that the necessary skills to use the system are already present and the finance is available to purchase and implement the package but that there is internal competition for the financial resource and that current hardware is outmoded and will need replacing before the package can be introduced.

This small example reveals some of the issues which can be uncovered by the carrying out of an internal audit.

Step four: identifying opportunities and threats

Having identified the significant issues, the manager can proceed to the identification of opportunities and threats. It is crucial at this stage to examine both internal and external factors to identify which significant issues arising from the audit will

The contribution of business planning

Table 4.1 Example of the use of SWOT

Internal issues		External issues	
Strengths	Weaknesses	Opportunities	Threats
Finance Staff skills in elderly care		Finance	Declining elderly population in the designated area
	Non-mental health unit	Health authority focus on mental health requirements	

present opportunities or constitute real threats to the aim in question. The manager can employ SWOT as in Table 4.1, where the aim in question is to consider opening a new unit for the elderly in a particular part of the city. This simple example aims to show that while the unit has the necessary finance and skills to carry out the plan, external factors indicate that it will not meet with the required support: the area being considered shows a demographic drop in the client group and the health authority's strategy is clearly focused on the needs of the mental health sector. In this situation the manager would be well advised to think again.

Carrying out PEST and SWOT analyses can be a lengthy process. However, time spent at this stage can save the organisation a significant amount of time and money and limit the risk of failure.

Research activities: how to obtain the information

A number of research methods are available to managers in undertaking PEST and SWOT analyses. Broadly these can be classified as primary and secondary data sources. Primary data are defined as both quantitative and qualitative information that is not already in existence. Secondary data are those that exist already (Box 4.7).

Carrying out some of the activities designed to produce primary data will provide the manager not only with 'hard' information but will also have the benefit of involving staff – and potential users of the service – in the discussions (and thereby enhancing their contribution), and provide other options for consideration in achieving the goal by involving a wider audience in the thinking.

Delivering the business

Box 4.7 Primary and secondary data sources

Primary data sources

Experiment:	Testing out the idea in a given area
Observation:	As participant or non-participant
Questioning:	
Quantitative methods:	Structured interview by questionnaire/surveys
	Self-administered interview
	Semi-structured interview
	Critical incident interview
	Diary keeping
	Telephone interview
	Open-ended interview
Qualitative methods:	Discussion/focus groups
	Brainstorming
	Delphi survey
	Judgemental method (i.e. informed opinion of experienced personnel)

Secondary data sources

Internal documentation:	Annual reports
	Human resource data
	Activity/trend profiles
	Performance indicators
	Financial data
External documentation:	Literature search
	Competitor activity
	Central and local Government reports

Step five: defining objectives

Having obtained the relevant information in relation to the aim, the manager is now in a position to:

- determine the likely success of the plan and consider various options in relation to achieving the aim,
- develop an outline business case showing the rationale and planned outcomes,
- develop objectives for implementing the plan, and
- develop scenarios or contingency plans by applying the 'what if …' principle.

The contribution of business planning

STRUCTURE OF THE PLAN

Rationale

This should be presented in the form of a statement outlining the goal: it should demonstrate its relation to the corporate mission or purpose, the current situation defining its relevance (by using information from the PEST and SWOT analyses), the planned outcome and a summary of the methods to be used to achieve that outcome as in:

- Where are we now?
- Where do we want to get to?
- How do we get there?
- And what resources will be required to achieve this?

Objectives

Following the description of the rationale, the principal objectives can be clearly stated. These should be SMART, i.e. Specific and simple (easy to comprehend), Measurable (i.e. phrased in terms of outcomes or results), Achievable (and agreed) (i.e. should be demanding but not impossible and agreed between relevant agencies), Realistic (should be explicit about constraints) and Time-related (should identify target dates and milestones).

An example of a SMART objective is: 'To open an extension to the elderly care unit in the Anyshire region by 30 April 2001 within a budget of £50 000.'

Operational planning

Having defined the rationale and principal objective in relation to the goal, the manager can proceed to develop an operational plan for implementation of the goal. These should follow the SMART principle. The application of marketing techniques is useful when establishing the operational plan to ensure that all areas are considered when objectives are defined. This can be summarised as deciding: Who, What, When, How, How much and Where?

In this situation, the six Ps used when developing marketing plans are a useful checklist. Areas to consider when developing operational objectives are:

Delivering the business

- *Product*   (i.e. the service being developed) What is its purpose; how long will it last; who wants it; does anyone else offer it; what are the options for delivering this service?

- *Price*   What budget is available; have the costs been established; what income needs to be raised from the project; have the various options been costed?

- *Place*   Is the service accessible; do alterations need to be made to existing facilities; are the appropriate resources available; what investment is required?

- *Personnel*   Are the right staff in post; is training required for existing staff; are there any implications for grading; if staff need to be recruited, what is an appropriate timescale for this?

- *Process*   How effective will the organisational structure be in delivering the service; are the facilities appropriate?

- *Promotion*   In this situation, promotion can be looked at as *communication*: are internal communications effective in relation to the implementation and delivery of the service; what do people within the organisation and outside it need to know; are costs involved; what methods of communication are available; when do people need to know and how are they to be informed and involved?

It is at this stage that action plans and Gantt charts become useful in managing the project.

Contingency planning

Bearing in mind all that has been said earlier in the chapter in relation to planning, in a climate of uncertainty it is advisable for contingency plans to be drawn up at this stage. Properly defined as contingency is an event which may occur and may be outside the manager's control (e.g. hospital merger). Contingency planning seeks to anticipate these events and define a plan of action in the event of the contingency occurring.

Evaluation and control

Quality assurance mechanisms should be defined and agreed within the operational plan. It is useful at this stage to revisit

113

The contribution of business planning

Drucker's features of service management: intangibility, inseparability, variability and perishability, and to define systems to monitor performance against these features. Performance standards may be quantitative or qualitative and can include:

- measurement of success against the defined objectives: levels of activity, achievement of timescales, financial reports against budget;
- competitor activity (if relevant);
- staff and user feedback;
- staff appraisal systems, including performance targets.

The establishment of proper planning control mechanisms is essential in ensuring that targets are achieved. The process can be costly and time-consuming, however, and it is therefore important to agree the need, timing and content of performance reports. Exception reporting can be a useful tool in ensuring that only those issues which require corrective treatment are considered.

The planning and control process should be dynamic, enabling adjustments to be made to original objectives where necessary. It is at this stage that an emergent planning strategy is useful, allowing individual managers to adjust objectives in the light of performance management indicators or changing circumstances.

WHY PLANS FAIL

There are a number of reasons why plans fail, despite research, objective setting and control systems. These often relate to the human factor – the most difficult variable. The Chartered Institute of Marketing (CIM 1991) summarises reasons for failure as follows:

- Lack of knowledge or interest about the purpose and goals of the organisation, leading to duplication of effort, conflicts of interest or indeed irrelevance of the project.
- Unwillingness in a time of change for management to be committed to one set of objectives or demonstrating an unwillingness to respond to new circumstances.
- Fear of failure or criticism when targets are set; deliberately planning to achieve low results on the premise that the failure is thereby the less.

- Lack of confidence in the manager's own skills or those of senior management to deliver the required resources.
- Lack of communication; this applies throughout the entire process from lack of information about the external environment to non-involvement of staff working on the project.
- Inappropriate objectives as a result of lack of information.
- Failure to involve all stakeholders.
- Imposed plans where no discussion creates resentment and resistance.
- Individual goals at variance with corporate goals.
- Conflict between individuals which jeopardises the outcome.
- Lack of clarity about individual responsibilities.
- Failure of the monitoring and control systems.
- Failure to address issues revealed through quality monitoring mechanisms.
- External factors beyond the manager's control.

Clearly, many of these issues can be overcome by an effective communication strategy and effective leadership. All staff and users involved in the plan should participate to an appropriate degree in the planning process. Communication, both oral and written, at agreed intervals will provide the necessary two-way flow of information required by all parties and limit the risk of counter-communication (in the form of gossip and rumour). Appropriate education and training programmes, supported by an effective appraisal system, will diminish the risk of failure. A reward system can provide a powerful motivating force for overcoming resistance. It is crucial that the manager does not regard the plan as set in stone once objectives have been drawn up. A willingness to listen to staff and users, to continue to scan the horizon and receive new information and act accordingly, to adjust the plan on an on-going basis will enhance the probability of success and, moreover, do so in a climate of cooperation and commitment.

CONCLUSION

We have a health service environment in which managers are required to plan. The need to remain aware constantly of changes within that environment is crucial to the success of any new initiative or the maintenance of a current service. The main points are that managers should:

The contribution of business planning

- be constantly aware of the political and social environment in which they operate;
- develop an understanding of the intangibles around service delivery which will help to deliver effective and efficient services;
- recognise the need to operate within the context of the organisation as a whole;
- understand the difficulties of formal planning in a climate of change or uncertainty;
- recognise the significance of staff and user involvement in planning and implementing new initiatives;
- comprehend the crucial importance of communication in successful planning;
- understand the importance of the human factor in management;
- recognise the necessity of regularly reviewing objectives and adjusting for changing circumstances; and
- establish effective performance measurement and information retrieval systems.

References

Brooks I, Weatherston J (1997) The business environment, challenges and changes. Hemel Hempstead: Prentice-Hall.

CIM Diploma (1991) Marketing planning and controls. London: BPP Publishing.

Cowell D W (1984) The marketing of services. Oxford: Heinemann.

Drucker P (1990) Managing the non-profit organisation. Oxford: Butterworth-Heinemann.

Hatch M J (1997) Organisation theory: modern symbolic and postmodern perspectives. New York: Oxford University Press.

Johns G, Scholes K (1997) Exploring corporate strategy, 4th edn. Hemel Hempstead: Prentice-Hall.

Johnson R (1990) The 24 hour business plan. London: Hutchinson Business Books.

Kotler P (1991) Marketing management: analysis, planning, implementation and control. Hemel Hempstead: Prentice-Hall.

Lawton A, Rose A (1994) Organisation and management in the public sector, 2nd edn. London: Pitman.

Further reading

Arjenti J (1980) Practical corporate planning. London: Allen & Unwin.

Department of Health (1998) Our healthier nation: a contract for health. London: The Stationery Office.

Robbins S (1997) Managing today. Hemel Hempstead: Prentice-Hall.

Delivering the business

Application 4:1

The plan to provide health care services in 1999/2000

The Plan to provide health care services in 1999/2000

SCUNTHORPE + GOOLE
hospitals n.h.s. trust

Application 4.1 is the Executive Summary of the Scunthorpe & Goole Hospitals NHS Trust business plan for 1999/2000. Note the style of presentation; it is clear and concise, and free of jargon. The reader can glean easily the clinical services the Trust provides, the services that are in place to support the clinical activity and the financial plans that will enable this to go ahead. Note also the references to agendas common to all NHS organisations, such as the comparative performance data review, the increased pressures in winter and the year 2000 preparations.

FOREWORD (BY CANDY MORRIS, CHIEF EXECUTIVE)

The UK government's plans to modernise the NHS have included a number of initiatives, but perhaps one of the most important is that described in the consultation paper 'A First Class Services: Quality in the New NHS'. The government's aim is to develop an NHS where there is fair access to consistently high-quality health care for all patients. Clinical governance is a key part of this concerted 10-year programme of work to improve the quality of patient care.

I am delighted that this emphasis is now being placed at the heart of patient care. Within the Trust we have developed our approach to this vital issue and expect to see our current drive to provide effective, efficient and caring services, reinforced by this initiative.

In this and other areas of work, we will continue to operate in partnership with Health Authorities, Primary Care Groups, social services, voluntary organisations and others. We seek to provide together, services which are integrated, effective and deal holistically with the needs of patients. Within this plan we have set ourselves a wide range of targets of the year, key amongst these being to balance our drive for high-quality and developing services with the need to maintain financial balance.

Finally, reference is made in this booklet to the crucial importance that staff play in delivering plans and targets. 1998/1999 was a successful year which demonstrated that our people are committed to the best interests of their patients and to the Trust. 1999/2000 will be equally demanding and I believe will be equally successful. I shall do my best to ensure our staff have opportunities to develop their potential and contribution to this organisation. This is the key to success.

INTRODUCTION

We are facing a number of challenges as the Millennium approaches and just a few of these are set out here:

- the reduction of waiting lists and waiting times,
- maintaining access to emergency care at all times,
- introducing clinical governance, an approach to improving the quality of clinical services,
- managing year 2000 issues,
- achieving financial balance,
- contributing to the Health Improvement Programme for South Humber and East Riding Health,
- developing close and effective links with the new Primary Care Groups,

- implementing the national information technology strategy and the national human resources framework,
- implementing the final round of proposals contained in the South Humber Health Review, and
- meeting a range of recommended service criteria based on, for example, minimum staffing, activity and population levels.

This plan aims to successfully meet each of these and the other challenges that confront us over the coming year.

We have set ourselves core objectives and have planned changes and improvements to our services, the great majority of which will be funded within current resources.

Core objectives

Our core objectives are to:

- Position and shape the Trust to play an effective role in the changing local NHS environment under 'The New NHS' agenda.
- Contribute towards the improvement of the general health of the population reducing inequalities and recognising the influence of social and economic factors in addition to health care.
- Manage all resources in a cost-effective manner to ensure the delivery of patient services which demonstrate value for money and which achieve and maintain the financial viability of the Trust.
- Work with commissioners to offer fair access to local health services in relation to people's needs.
- Ensure that the local delivery of health care is effective, appropriate and timely with the aim of continually improving service quality.
- Ensure that local service delivery remains sensitive to the needs of the individual by focusing on the patient and carer view of the quality of treatment and care they receive.
- Contribute to improvements in the health of the local population by focusing on the clinical outcomes of packages of care and evaluating their effectiveness
- Maximise the use of Goole and District Hospital and develop a strategy to maintain the level of utilisation in support of the provision of local health care.

Business plan – Scunthorpe & Goole Hospitals NHS Trust

119

● Continue to recognise the key role of our staff in the delivery of health improvement and further develop their potential, contribution and commitment to improve overall performance.

In all of this our staff are the key to success and we will continue to pay special attention to their individual development.

We will continue to operate in a spirit of partnership with all local health and social care agencies to deliver these objectives. Indeed, to meet the criteria for service accreditation and for other reasons, clinical and financial, the South Bank health care organisations will work to develop a strategy for the way ahead for South Humber. This must take into account all the issues including a review of clinical service configuration and also, possibly the configuration of organisations on the South Bank.

THE TRUST

Scunthorpe & Goole Hospitals NHS Trust, established on 1 April 1993, provides a broad and expanding range of in-patient, day case and outpatient services. These are provided across the medical and surgical specialties supported by clinical and non-clinical services, largely through the two hospitals in Scunthorpe and Goole, but also in the community. The major purchaser continues to be South Humber Health Authority although, with the development of Primary Care Groups leading to the establishment of Primary Care Trusts, the majority of the purchasing decisions will soon be made by these bodies.

IMPROVING PATIENT SERVICES

In 1999/2000, we aim to make a number of service improvements and some of these are set out here.

Involvement in Health Improvement Programmes

We will ensure full and effective involvement in the development of programmes, especially those for cancer, diabetes, people with heart disease and stroke, teenage conception and elderly people. We will also contribute to the development of Joint Investment Plans.

Inpatient/day service, rehabilitation unit

A revised model of rehabilitation will be implemented, primarily for stroke patients and patients with neurological problems, in a combined, purpose-designed, inpatient and day unit.

Critical care

An in-house haemofiltration service will be developed, funded from charitable sources, which will prevent some patients having to travel to other hospitals.

Intensive care unit staffing will be arranged to ensure that at any one time, there can be the equivalent of three intensive care beds and one high-dependency bed in use.

Cancer services

Accreditation for breast and colorectal cancer is a priority. Effective preparation will be made for the revisit in October of the Accreditation Team. Accreditation will also be sought as required for other specialties such as gynaecology and head and neck cancer.

We will continue to support the development of inpatient palliative care beds at Lindsey Lodge Hospice.

Improved performance

We will continue to work closely with GPs and others to reduce to national average rates the number of patients that are referred to hospital, especially where they can be effectively cared for in the community. We will also seek to increase the number of people treated as day cases and reduce the numbers of days people stay in hospital so they can go home as soon as they are well enough. Doing all this will result in the closure by March 2000 of a medical ward at Scunthorpe General Hospital, in fulfilment of the South Humber review recommendations.

Support to tackle winter pressures

The winter peak in demand for health care services is recognised to be a multiagency issue. Social services and acute, community and primary health care services collaborate in order to help reduce pressure on hospital services. This has been achieved in the past through a range of innovative projects and an ability to access resources to place patients appropriately outside acute services. It is intended to adopt a similar approach for the winter 1999/2000.

Child and family services

We are keen to pursue the integration of acute and community child health services. Within the field of gynaecology the development of an endometrial ablation service is being considered with an aim to move more inpatient work to day case and day case work to outpatients.

We will also look at the possibility of establishing a 'post menopausal bleed' clinic, by altering existing clinic arrangements.

A midwifery centre will be developed in Brigg and a replacement ultrasound system, costing in excess of £100 000 will be purchased.

Professions allied to medicine

We aim to begin providing occupational therapy in the accident & emergency department and a 7-day therapy service in the new rehabilitation unit, in partnership with other professionals within the multidisciplinary team.

Through the Joint Investment Plans a collaborative therapy service will continue to be developed in conjunction with the Community Trust, Primary Care and the local authority. Through the Health Improvement Programme for Diabetes it will be possible to appoint a second chiropodist.

Diagnostic and therapeutic services

A business case for remote order communications will be developed to involve pathology and medical imaging

Delivering the business

requests and drugs prescribing. This will be a bid against the government's modernisation fund. Other developments include establishing a local magnetic resonance imaging (MRI) service on a cost neutral basis and automating the blood transfusion service.

Services at Goole

We shall continue to work towards the fullest use of Goole & District Hospital. Plans for the increased provision of primary, community and secondary care will be developed wherever possible.

The acquired brain injury unit on ward 4 will open and full support will be given to the development of a Healthy Living Centre for Goole. We hope also to replace parts of the X-ray equipment.

We will work with the East Riding of Yorkshire and North Lincolnshire Councils to facilitate improved transport services between Scunthorpe and Goole.

Medical staffing

Consultant staff will be recruited for those areas where vacancies exist.

Urology

Appointment to a collaborative arrangement possibly with Hull and Grimsby.

Oral/maxillofacial

Appointment to a collaborative arrangement with Hull and Grimsby.

Rheumatology

Sessions provided from North East Lincolnshire NHS Trust.

Medicine

Post 1 with an interest in respiratory medicine, post 2 with an interest in elderly medicine.

Business plan – Scunthorpe & Goole Hospitals NHS Trust

Dermatology

Appointment to an agreed service model with the Royal Hallamshire Hospital, Sheffield.

Communication with other providers and commissioners of health care services

We will establish firm links with North Lincolnshire and other Primary Care Groups (PCGs) to ensure that our services continue to meet the requirements of those who commission them.

Waiting lists

In total 4537 patients were waiting for a hospital procedure at the end of March 1999, against a target of 4810 (273 better than target). By the end of 1998/1999 the number of patients waiting had reduced by 25.5%. Plans are in place to achieve further reductions in waiting times for inpatient and day case procedures and to reduce the number of patients waiting over 13 weeks for first routine outpatient appointment to March 1998 levels.

Capital programme

We shall be investing almost £2 million in purchasing medical and surgical equipment and in other capital development – in support of improved patient services.

Patient services

The range of treatments and minor operative procedures provided within the outpatient environment will be expanded. Bed management initiatives will continue, including the management of winter pressures, emergency admissions and waiting lists, ensuring effective bed utilisation. We will also provide an enhanced medical records service, extending opening hours for casenote location and provision.

EFFECTIVE HEALTH CARE

The new NHS expects its organisations to continuously improve the quality of their services. Clinical governance is central to this strategy. A Clinical Governance Steering Group will be working to bring together many of the structures already in place, leading to the production of a first annual report in April 2000. The group will assess the current status of systems in place and develop an Action Plan to address areas where further progress can be made.

The Departments of Postgraduate Medical Education (PGME) and Effective Health Care play a vital role in the process. The PGME department provides education and training facilities that are available to all staff. Increasing use of information technology will further enhance access to information. The Effective Health Care Department supports the provision of evidence-based, clinically effective services. It enables a system of clinical performance management, using national and local audit, benchmarking and clinical indicators. The department undertakes patient satisfaction monitoring, seeks to implement the findings of quality surveys and encourages research and development.

The approach of the Trust to clinical governance will bring together many aspects of its current work to produce a culture of continuous improvement and thus to safeguard high standards to care.

FINANCIAL PLANS

The Trust achieved a small surplus for 1998/1999, against the target required to break even. This is a £1.2 million improvement on the previous year and a £600 000 improvement on the original rolling plan. This substantial achievement has been attained through delivery of the first 2 years of the Trust's 3-year recovery plan, which identified a range of actions to reduce costs of services and improve the use of our hospital sites. We therefore commence 1999/2000 with a balanced financial plan, but this does include a cost improvement programme of £2.6 million. We have also contributed with other Health Agencies to the achievement of non-recurrent financial balance for South Humber as a whole for 1999/2000.

Business plan – Scunthorpe & Goole Hospitals NHS Trust

All this means careful use of our resources and, in particular, the phasing of our capital programme. We will seek to make the best of opportunities presented by the modernisation fund to enhance service delivery. In particular, our proposals will build on current expertise and local partnership arrangements.

We will bid for NHS modernisation funds for improvements to the following services:

- *Lung cancer* Bid for second physician in respiratory medicine.
- *Accident & Emergency* Improvements to the A&E Department.
- *Diabetes* Bid to extend the current diabetes centre.
- *Diagnostic and therapeutic services* Remote order communication.

HUMAN RESOURCES – MANAGEMENT AND DEVELOPMENT

Our priority will be to ensure that all staff are able to make the best possible contribution, individually and collectively, to the Trust's objectives, values and performance. In this way we will improve health and patient care and our contribution to the wider local health agenda. Priorities aimed at developing staff potential, contribution and commitment consistent with the national human resources framework include:

- Internal and patch wide organisational and management development to support cultural, organisational and service changes including comprehensive clinical governance and the local Health Improvement Programme.
- Staff partnership and involvement improvements, particularly those recommended by the 1998/99 staff working group including a staff attitude survey, and a robust internal communications focus.
- Sharing (where appropriate) scarce specialist support services, expertise and skills in pursuance of South Humber Health Authority's review recommendations.
- Robust staff planning to minimise millennium disruption to services.

- Continuing development of robust recruitment strategies for scarce skill areas.
- Progression of the Trust's medical staffing strategy and accreditation, in collaboration with other organisations.
- Progression of equality of opportunity, family-friendly good practice and workplace health and staff support strategies, to enhance the quality of staff working life, health and workforce diversity.
- Completion of the third year of the Investors in People development plan and the seeking of re-accreditation.
- Collaboration with local education consortium colleagues to develop a robust, integrated human resources plan to supply and train staff to meet service needs, including the Health Improvement Programme.
- Smooth implementation of new employment legislation and national pay system changes.

YEAR 2000

The Trust has based its service continuity plans around a possible five-fold increase in activity over the millennium period. These plans will ensure that high-quality services remain available during periods of high demand. The Trust has revised its major incident plans in light of the millennium, the anticipated additional workload and the possibility of technical failures in the community, including major utilities such as power and communication systems. Equipment and internal system compliance was tested in 1998/99 and non-compliant items have been either made compliant or replaced. The ability of both Scunthorpe and Goole Hospitals to function using locally generated power has been tested. Continuity plans will be tested before the end of October 1999.

IT AND INFORMATION SERVICES

The publication of the new NHS Information Strategy, 'Information for Health', gives a clear remit to deliver on key programmes and initiatives. Our priorities are to:

Business plan – Scunthorpe & Goole Hospitals NHS Trust

- Work under the control and management of the Year 2000 Project Board to ensure that the Trust will be able to function over the millennium period.
- Put in place an appropriate plan to ensure that in the event of a disaster, appropriate contingencies can be effected to recover critical services and systems supported by the department.
- Continue to work on the Clinical Health Record Information System (CHRIS) project to develop appropriate solutions and systems to support the delivery of clinical information.
- Ensure that the use of web and browser technology plays a significant role in the delivery of clinical information across the Trust.
- Develop the clinical nursing information system.
- Continue the work to upgrade the Trust-wide network and desktop infrastructure.
- Put in place the necessary infrastructure to adequately train clinicians and other users.
- Continue opportunities for joint working to be assessed as part of the development to support the local information strategy.

ESTATES AND SUPPORT SERVICES

Financial constraints impose an approach which aims to improve efficiency and rationalise services and estate where appropriate. The following developments will be implemented in 1999/2000:

- The improvement of transport arrangements between Scunthorpe and Goole.
- The development of partnership arrangements with other organisations within and outside the NHS.
- The introduction of changes to patient transport quality targets.
- The revision of arrangements for estates management and staff development.
- Improvements to the utilisation of estates accommodation.
- Improvements to equipment utilisation.
- The management of the estate and support services elements of the capital programme.

MONITORING PERFORMANCE

It is important to know whether we are succeeding against the many targets and goals set for 1999/2000. There are a number of ways in which performance is monitored through the year. These include review of progress each month by the Board and the Corporate Management Team and within divisional teams.

In addition, performance against service level agreements will be reviewed with the Primary Care Groups and Health Authorities and performance against the South Humber Performance Management Agreement will be reviewed with all the organisations involved.

COMPARATIVE PERFORMANCE DATA REVIEW

Figures 4.1.1–4.1.3 provide a useful comparison of Trust performance compared with national targets.

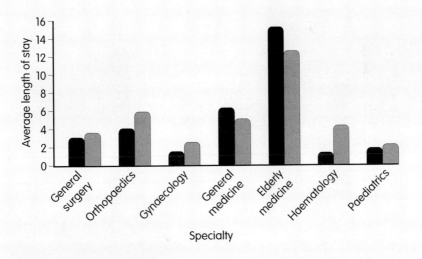

■ Current average length of stay

■ Target length of stay

Figure 4.1.1 Comparative performance data review: average length of stay.

129

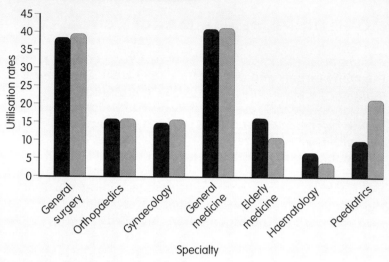

■ Current utilisation rate

■ Target length of stay

Figure 4.1.2 Comparative performance data review: utilisation rates.

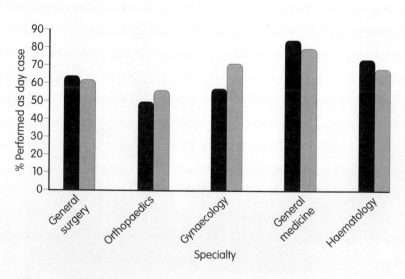

■ Current day case %

■ Target %

Figure 4.1.3 Comparative performance data review: day case rates.

Delivering the business

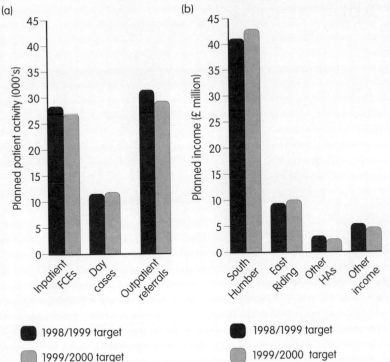

Figure 4.1.4 Comparative performance data review: (a) planned patient activity, (b) planned income.

Figure 4.1.4 shows the level of income we expect from each purchaser and the level of activity we intend to provide.

YOUR VIEWS ARE WELCOME

If you have any comments or queries about this summary, or the services provided by the Trust, please contact: Candy Morris, Chief Executive, Scunthorpe & Goole Hospitals NHS Trust, Scunthorpe General Hospital, Cliff Gardens, Scunthorpe, North Lincolnshire DN15 7BH. Telephone: (01724) 290147, Facsimile: (01724) 282427. Email: Candy.Morris@sgh-tr.trent.nhs.uk

Reproduced from 'The Plan to provide health care services in 1999/2000' with permission of Scunthorpe & Goole Hospitals NHS Trust.

Leeds Health Improvement Programme

Leeds Health Improvement Programme

tackling health inequalities in Leeds

information leaflet

Application 4.2 is a summary of the Leeds Health Improvement Programme (HImP). This is a 3-year plan of action for improving health, reducing inequalities and for delivering better health and social care for the people of Leeds. The document demonstrates how the principles and processes of business planning are useful and appropriate to apply in a range of management contexts.

HEALTH IMPROVEMENT PROGRAMME 1999/2002

The Health Improvement Programme is a 3-year plan of action for improving health, reducing inequalities and delivering better health and social care. It covers:

- the most important needs of the local population and how these are to be met,
- the main health and social care requirements of local people and how local services should be developed to meet them,
- the range, location and investment required in services to meet the health needs of local people.

Delivering the business

The Health Improvement Programme has been drawn up by Leeds Health Authority in partnership with other agencies including Leeds City Council, Voluntary Action Leeds, Leeds Community Health Council, the NHS Trusts and Primary Care Groups.

The Programme is based on the following principles:

- Everyone should have the same chance of good health no matter who they are and where they live.
- Organisations whose decisions can affect people's health should work together to improve health.
- The public should have a say in these decisions.

The Health Improvement Programme reflects the health, social care and joint strategies within the city and translates them into practice. It also demonstrates a commitment to Leeds Initiative's 'Vision for Leeds'.

The first Health Improvement Programme is to be updated annually with contributions from a much wider group of partners and the local people.

We are committed to working towards improving the quality of life for the people of Leeds as we move into the next millennium.

The Health Improvement Programme identifies the following priorities for action.

Health needs assessment

- Agreeing priorities and ways to build a picture of health inequalities in Leeds

Influences on health

- Developing partnerships to improve health
- Improving the health of those in society with the most need
- Removing barriers to employment and opportunity
- Improving the environment
- Encouraging greater use of public transport and increasing walking and cycling
- Improving the quality of housing
- Reducing crime and disorder to create better neighbourhoods

Leeds Health Improvement Programme

- Making good quality affordable food more accessible
- Increasing the opportunities for young people to be more physically active
- Developing access to services for minority ethnic groups
- Involving local people to address the concerns of communities.

Health topics

- Reducing deaths from heart disease
- Improving the quality, effectiveness and speed of access to cancer services
- Reducing accident rates among disadvantaged groups
- Improving the mental health of the population
- Improving treatment for people with mental health problems
- Taking local action on drug misuse, alcohol and smoking
- Providing information and support on sexual health
- Developing partnerships for improving health in the home
- Tackling violence against women and children
- Developing a health promoting schools award
- Establishing a city-wide forum on health in the workplace.

Health and social care services

- Developing services which help older people to be independent and healthy
- Developing better services for children, including providing more in the local community.
- Reducing waiting times and waiting lists for hospital treatment
- Developing primary and community services to improve their quality and convenience.

LEEDS AS A 'HEALTH ACTION ZONE'

Leeds became a Health Action Zone in April 1999 and this work will link closely with the Health Improvement Programme. The Health Action Zone focuses on action to tackle the root causes of ill health, deliver better services and remove barriers to working together. An action plan identifying programmes of work has been developed. Key themes include:

- Improving health through partnerships
- Delivering better services
- Community development and involvement
- Healthy living
- Ethnicity and health
- Health improving information.

NEXT STEPS – PLAN OF ACTION

The Health Improvement Programme will be developed over time to produce a more comprehensive document by 2002.

This first document is based on jointly agreed city-wide strategies and policies. The second stage will involve local communities. This means coordinating community involvement with other agencies in particular linking with the city council's community planning process and the voluntary and community sector initiative and the Primary Care Groups.

Primary Care Groups will also make a significant contribution to the development of the next Health Improvement Programme. They will use their new roles and responsibilities to feed the local perspective into future programmes. This next stage will involve:

- the public
- academic institutions
- voluntary agencies
- the independent sector
- criminal justice agencies
- training institutions
- commercial sector
- staff organisations.

TIMETABLE OF EVENTS

- Launch   July 1999
- Themed events   September 1999

Leeds Health Improvement Programme

	December 1999
	March 2000
● Community involvement	July–November 1999
● Draft of second Programme starts	September 1999

For further copies of the information leaflet, the Summary document or the full Health Improvement Programme, please contact: Christine Burnett at Leeds Health Authority, Blenheim House, West One, Duncombe Street, Leeds, LS1 4PL. Also available on our website: www.leedshealth.org.uk

Reproduced from 'Leeds Health Improvement Programme' with permission from Leeds Health Authority.

Delivering the business

Application 4:3 *Jill Ellison*

Emergency admissions – understanding the problem

Application 4.3 recounts, retrospectively, how engaging in joint planning initiatives helped address the challenge of increased winter emergency admissions in one Trust.

Emergency admissions during the winter period are rising and have become one of the main challenges facing the health service today. This has not gone unnoticed by both recent governments. Only weeks after being elected, the then secretary of state for health, Frank Dobson, wrote to all Health Authorities, Trusts and Social Service Departments stating 'the first priority above all others, is to make adequate provision for emergency care'. A short time later he made the famous Berlin Wall analogy, referring to the barriers that exist between health and social care and the need for the two to work in partnership if the NHS is to tackle these difficult issues.

The challenge is for hospitals, community care providers and social services to work together and respond to this growth in demand and to manage emergency admissions in such a way as to avoid what is seen increasingly as a winter crisis.

CHARACTERISTICS OF EMERGENCY ADMISSIONS

There is general agreement regarding the epidemiology of emergency admissions and increasing recognition that a multiagency approach is essential.

- Admissions peak, usually between December and February.
- Admission rates vary, but tend to be highest in areas of greatest deprivation and where a high proportion of the population are 65 years of age and above.
- Growth is higher in medical rather than surgical conditions and in particular, diseases of the respiratory, cardiovascular and nervous systems.
- Only approximately half of the patients admitted are referred by a GP.
- Accident and emergency departments act as gatekeepers, and from here patients are more easily processed into the hospital rather than back into the community.

Primary care provision is crucial, as there are wide variations in GP practice and community nursing services. Equally, effective discharge planning is essential and this must commence at the point of admission, if not before.

WHAT DOES THIS MEAN FOR HEARTLANDS AND SOLIHULL HOSPITALS?

Birmingham Heartlands Hospital is the larger of two hospitals in the Trust. Heartlands is a 900-bedded teaching hospital, situated on the east side of the city, serving a population of 267 000. Unlike the sister hospital based in Solihull, there are the inner city problems of social deprivation, such as poor housing and high unemployment. There is an above average minority ethnic population and the over 65 years group accounts for only 15% of the population but for 54% of the medical emergency admissions.

Every year has seen a year on year growth in emergency admissions of approximately 4%. Figure 4.3.1 shows the

Delivering the business

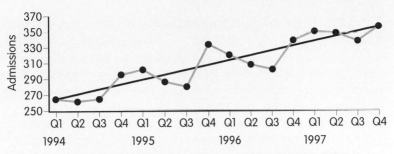

Time period (calendar year quarters) Jan 1994–Dec 1997

Figure 4.3.1 Average weekly medical admissions per quarter for Heartlands and Solihull Hospitals.

pattern of emergency admissions during the period January 1994 to December 1997 across both hospitals.

THE WINTER OF 1996/97 – THE CHAIN OF EVENTS

Local control plans were implemented in 1996 with the intention of averting any possible winter crisis. The overall outcome for Birmingham was not inconsistent with the national picture in that, as anticipated, winter pressures were greater than the previous year, but the situation was helped in that the spells of icy weather were limited and there were no epidemics of influenza. However, notwithstanding these favourable features, hospitals were placed under severe strain for a third winter running. There was also serious disruption to the normal delivery of both emergency and elective care and a consequential effect on the quality of patient care and staff morale.

Specific problems identified included:

- Lack of additional beds and flexi wards.
- The availability of nursing staff in terms of number and skills to staff. The availability of support staff such as social workers to effect timely delays and discharges as the demand rose.
- The lack of availability of accurate and timely bed information.
- Variations in daily admission and discharge patterns.
- The build up of patients in A&E during periods of peak demand, leading to trolley waits.

Emergency admissions

LESSONS LEARNT FROM 1996/97

The most important action was to establish a post-winter working group to identify all the measures required to manage winter admission pressures. This was underpinned by a new understanding that anything less than a fully integrated, collaborative approach involving both health and social care professionals would fail. This is referred to as a whole system approach and looks at the interaction of pressures around emergency care, hospital discharge and the availability of care in the community. There are seven stages:

Stage 1   Pre-admission
Stage 2   Admission to hospital
Stage 3   Treatment
Stage 4   Assessment
Stage 5   Rehabilitation and recovery
Stage 6   Hospital discharge
Stage 7   Continuing care and re-admission.

At each point it is possible to identify: the decision points concerned, factors (pressures/incentives) affecting the decision, factors/interventions likely to improve outcomes, indicators of system failure/success (e.g. re-admission rates), costs of improving outcomes (e.g. target resources) and benefits of improving outcomes (e.g. reduced admissions).

By using this framework it was possible to identify a series of actions requiring multiagency, cross-boundary collaboration. These were detailed in a comprehensive report, 'The A–Z of Winter Pressures', prepared in house, which was made available to everyone in the organisation, and also to the community and social services. Examples from this are given in Box 4.3.1.

THE IMPACT OF THE MULTISYSTEM APPROACH

As predicted, the winter of 1997/98 was as busy as previous years with many hospitals experiencing a new peak in admissions. There were, however, a few notable differences:

● The winter peak in admissions occurred later, thought to be due to the milder weather experienced.

Box 4.3.1 Examples of good practice initiatives implemented

1. **Pre-admission**
   - Two rapid response teams were established in the community, to be used by GPs to refer patients requiring more intensive nursing care at home, with the aim of avoiding admission
   - The additional purchase of nursing home beds for GP access
   - A public health incentive to encourage wider uptake of the influenza vaccine

2. **Admission to hospital**
   - The introduction of an out-of-hours GP scheme within the A&E Department. This acted as an effective gatekeeper, ensuring other alternatives to admission are activated
   - Training given to A&E nursing staff to enhance their skills in triage, thereby reducing waiting times.

3. **Treatment**
   In response to the need to provide rapid and effective treatment several clinically focused changes were made:
   - The introduction of a multidisciplinary single patient record
   - The identification of an acute medical physician to take daily responsibility for coordinating activities in A&E and initiating additional ward rounds
   - The immediate transfer of all patients over 75 years of age to the care of the on-call and acute facilities within the elderly care service

4. **Assessment**
   - Additional social workers were made available to support the comprehensive assessment and discharge planning process
   - Emergency assessments were undertaken in the community
   - An enhanced home care service to provide emergency and temporary assistance in the home was developed

5. **Rehabilitation and recovery**
   - Step-down facilities were provided for patients who are past the acute phase of their illness but require an intermediate care bed before going home or moving to a community home placement

6. **Hospital discharge**
   - Introduction of multiagency discharge protocols which are closely monitored to ensure the discharge planning process starts at the point of admission, agreed targets are completed on time and an option of intermediate care considered for patients whose discharge is delayed
   - A discharge lounge facility introduced for suitable patients awaiting discharge in line with agreed protocols

Emergency admissions

Box 4.3.1 Cont'd

7. Continuing care and re-admission
- The elderly care directorate established a scheme, staffed by hospital health care professionals, which would provide specialist support in the community to patients discharged home or in step-down facilities
- Re-admissions hotline established

- There was less disruption to elective admissions and many hospitals even managed to reduce waiting lists.
- There was limited negative media coverage and greater public confidence.

In the organisation there was a real spirit of everyone working together and a feeling that the pressures were being managed actively.

The major task ahead is to evaluate the initiatives implemented to improve our understanding of both the reasons for the increases in winter admissions and also the actions which have the greatest impact on reducing admissions and managing discharges effectively. This is no mean feat. However, the issues are complex and cross both health and social care boundaries and as such require a fully integrated and collaborative approach in order that a seamless, fluent service is experienced by the patients.

Delivering the business

Chapter **Five**

The human resource in business planning

- **Part 1: Planning for change**
  Steve Gosling, Helen Fields
  Supporting the workforce
  The implications for NHS
  organisations
  The contribution of
  human resource
  management

- **Part 2: Workforce planning**
  Carol Wilby
  Workforce planning through
  the 1990s
  Workforce planning – the
  theory
  Workforce planning – the
  reality

OVERVIEW

In Chapter 4 Linda Terry described and discussed the value of a business plan to managers in health care, and we looked at some examples of business plans to see how the principles can be applied in different contexts. Chapter 5, which is in two parts, builds upon Chapter 4 and looks at the human element in the process of business planning. In Part 1, Steve Gosling and Helen Fields look at the changing pattern of work, and how organisational change influences the workforce in terms of both the organisational need and the career opportunities for staff.

In Part 2, Carol Wilby describes the workforce planning process, a specific form of business planning which makes the link between the business of the organisation and the education and training needs of the staff. The forward planning element is important here, as the 'roll in' time in preparing health professionals for practice is substantial when one takes into account the recruitment phase and the actual education process. Thus, in this changing world, the workforce plans made now may not be such a 'good fit' in 3–4 years' time.

PART 1: PLANNING FOR CHANGE (STEVE GOSLING, HELEN FIELDS)

Supporting the workforce

The nature of personal and organisational development in the NHS is characterised by a number of contextual factors – factors that impact upon both public and private sector organisations. To say that the 1990s was a period of rapid and far reaching organisational change in the NHS is an understatement. We have seen the creation of NHS Trusts and changing roles for Health Authorities, the creation and abolition of Family Health Service Authorities, the reduction in the number of Regional Health Authorities and their transition into smaller/fewer regional offices of the NHS Executive, the establishment of general practitioner fundholding, the disestablishment of general practitioner fundholding, the introduction of Primary Care Groups – the list seems endless.

Organisational change has been accompanied by shifts in the way that services are planned, commissioned and delivered. For example, we have seen the increasing emphasis on community and primary care as the focus of both purchasing and delivery of patient care, the establishment of the internal market with its emphasis on competition and the growth of 'consumerism', alongside attempts to place patients, carers and local communities at the core of the development and delivery of health care.

Furthermore, change will continue to be a feature of the NHS. The English White Paper, 'The New NHS: Modern, Dependable' (Department of Health 1997), signals the end of the 'internal market' and a period of further organisational change which will see NHS Trust mergers, significant changes to the role of Health Authorities and the establishment of Primary Care Groups and Primary Care Trusts. Also fundamental is the wider strategy for health contained in the government Green Paper 'Our Healthier Nation' (Department of Health 1998a), and the subsequent White

Paper 'Saving Lives: our Healthier Nation' (Department of Health 1999). Devolution is set to bring about further differences in organisational structure, but the general principles of human resource management are transferable within all four countries of the UK.

Organisational change has taken place (and will continue to take place) in the context of resource pressures and demands to reduce management costs. In line with the private sector we have witnessed the creation of smaller/slimmer organisations but with wider ranging responsibilities.

The development of what Charles Handy (1990) calls the 'Shamrock' organisation (one feature of which is a reduction in the number of core staff directly employed by the organisation) has been particularly significant for those working at middle management levels where the impact of these changes has been most acutely felt. A reduction in the number of middle management positions has created an organisational and experience gulf between the top and lower levels of management. How individuals are enabled to progress to senior positions continues to be a key challenge for management and leadership development in the NHS today.

Similarly, the loss of middle management positions in Health Authorities and Trusts means that the creation of opportunities for new entrants to management, e.g. those wishing to move from clinical posts or graduates wishing to enter the NHS from university, to gain experience at these levels is becoming more of a priority.

The organisational changes referred to have also required managers to acquire new and different skills, a trend further reinforced by the English White Paper 'The New NHS: Modern, Dependable' and by the sister White Papers of Wales and Scotland, the Northern Ireland consultation papers discussed in Chapter 2 and the recently published NHS Plan (Department of Health 2000).

The following skills and abilities are likely to become essential prerequisites for the NHS manager and clinical professionals:

- networking and influencing abilities, with less reliance on directing and controlling skills;
- better understanding of organisational development tools and techniques to influence change and to develop new organisational styles and cultures;
- the ability to work collaboratively and develop partnerships across professional and organisational boundaries;

The human resource in business planning

145

● the development of skills to manage complexity and uncertainty.

Chapter 10 emphasises the need for effective multidisciplinary working, always a feature of the NHS. This will become increasingly important in the light of the governmental requirement that doctors and nurses become more centrally placed in the process of service planning and development, for example in the establishment and leadership of Primary Care Groups. The framework of clinical governance requires managers and clinicians to work closely together, understand different perspectives and find common ground, with a shared language, as the basis for joint action. Recruiting and developing managers from clinical backgrounds will contribute to the breakdown of some of the actual and perceived barriers that have existed in the past and will add to the pool of flexible and widely experienced managers required by the NHS.

Ironically, organisational fragmentation (between purchasers and providers, between different types of providers) has made the acquisition of skills and a breadth of experience gained through working in a variety of organisational settings more difficult to obtain. Developing managers from a variety of professional backgrounds and with wide experience in different organisations will have to be a managed and facilitated process rather than one left to individual employee or employer discretion. Smaller/flatter and fewer organisations, with the concomitant reduction in the number of posts available to NHS staff, has led to the breakdown of traditional career paths. The notion of a 'successful' career that is based on upward career progression has gone; the 'career ladder' has been replaced by the 'career climbing frame' (NHS Executive 1996). This may result in long periods in one job, horizontal (not vertical) career moves, frequent renewal of old or acquisition of new skills becoming the norm, but in order to make this work, attitudes towards processes of career development will begin to change.

The implications for NHS organisations

The old psychological contract between employer and employee, i.e. in return for employee loyalty employers offer a 'job for life', will need to be replaced by a new partnership contract, i.e. one where organisations offer employment security (not employment guarantees). This can be achieved by helping individuals to develop their skills and experience in ways that not only meet immediate employer requirements but also make the individuals more marketable in career terms and enhance their role flexibility and employability. Staff retention will be increasingly dependent upon employers honouring their side of this contract and providing a range of development opportunities, including not only training courses but also access to supported experience-based learning.

There now has to be a greater focus on the more flexible development of people with the appropriate skills and competencies to meet existing and future roles rather than on highly structured succession planning processes. This increased flexibility will need to be demonstrated in two ways:

1. in how staff are developed, through the increased use of a diverse range of development options such as structured secondments, shadowing, mentoring and access to multiprofessional training experiences;
2. in how individuals plan and progress their careers, with increasing emphasis being placed on a breadth of experience gained through lateral career moves rather than traditional vertical progression.

This will lead to skills and expertise being gained, as well as utilised in different organisational settings, such as the health service, local authority, voluntary and private sectors. The movement of staff across organisational boundaries will almost certainly become more commonplace as inter-organisational working partnerships become more established.

Defining the skills and competencies required in the future and then equipping staff with them will continue to be a key challenge for the NHS. This will require the close integration of personal development with the business objectives of the organisation. Important questions about the nature of the organisation in the future, the range and style of services it will have responsibility for and the concomitant implications for the number of staff, their skills and abilities will need to be addressed more systematically than at present. There will also need to be a closer partnership developed between employers and the higher education sector to ensure that those responsible for planning and delivering education and training remain in touch with changing service requirements.

Ensuring that staff can 'maximise their contribution' to shaping organisational change and development is a concept promoted by centre (i.e. government). However, the simplicity of these words conceals a fundamental challenge – that of creating

The human resource in business planning

and supporting a culture of lifelong learning throughout the workforce. This will be particularly important for those individuals who have been denied or excluded from opportunities to learn and/or who do not yet recognise their own potential and their own responsibilities to learn and contribute in meaningful ways.

Lifelong learning has been given greater legitimacy and urgency through the publication of the government Green Paper 'The Learning Age' (Department of Education and Employment 1998), and the subsequent White Paper 'Learning to Succeed' (Department of Education and Employment 1999). For the NHS to realise its significant power and potential as a leading edge employer this will mean (inter alia) putting in place flexible and stimulating workplace learning opportunities which are designed to unlock the potential and diversity of individuals and to harness this potential for the benefit of the organisation. This may range from ensuring that everyone in the organisation is helped to formulate and realise a personal development plan to establishing 'learning centres' within the workplace or in partnership with other organisations such as local authorities, Training and Enterprise Councils and the further education and higher education sectors.

It could be argued that the combined impetus of the policies put forward in 'The New NHS' and 'The Learning Age' provide the most challenging context for personal and organisational development in the NHS in the new millennium. There are also powerful messages here for the collective potential of the Regional Education Development Groups and Education and Training Consortia in England (discussed in Part 2 of this chapter), who are charged with developing longer term strategies for workforce planning, education and development. Such strategies will need to clearly align with the service delivery implications of local Health Improvement Plans. In addition, education commissioning, development and provision will increasingly be measured against more sophisticated quality benchmarks and performance management arrangements. This backdrop also illustrates the important role of Education and Training Consortia in extending their collaborative partnerships and commissioning potential at local level with Training and Enterprise Councils and, nationally, with relevant national training organisations, in realising the individual and organisational benefits of lifelong learning. Finally, whilst personal development must clearly have a beneficial impact on individuals (on their skills and abilities), the evaluation and demonstration of the long-term benefits to employers and organisations is vital if they are to continue investing in the development of their staff. Increasingly, employers will want to see tangible outcomes for their organisations, not only in increasing the range and quality of skills/talent available to them but also in improving the performance of the organisation.

Limited resources, changing organisational structures and new skill requirements will require that the NHS develops managers from all professional backgrounds who are skilled, flexible and equipped to deliver highly demanding clinical and managerial agendas. Individuals must also be supported to realise their own responsibilities for continuing professional development and lifelong learning. Personal development will increasingly be the outcome of a marriage of individual and organisational objectives assessed and delivered in partnership between staff and their employers.

The contribution of human resource management

Described above is the context of organisational change that has characterised and will continue to characterise the NHS in years to come – ability to change, responsiveness, adaptability, flexibility are features required of NHS organisations and the people they employ. Retaining the commitment of employees during periods of constant change to work content and methods requires sophisticated and sensitive approaches to management, backed up by a supportive human resources strategy, of which a commitment to personal development is a key feature.

Human resource management has a crucial contribution to play in ensuring that the NHS recruits, retains and develops staff who are equipped to perform the roles required of them both now and in the future. The NHS, as the single largest employer in Europe, cannot afford to ignore the connection between the management and development of those staff and the effectiveness of the organisation and the services it delivers. The Audit Commission (1997) in its report on staff retention in the NHS, highlighted the negative impact of poor people management practices and procedures. The Commission's study concluded that management practice was the most significant cause of differences in staff turnover between NHS Trusts, with a concomitant impact on teamworking, morale, quality of service, effectiveness and efficiency.

Indeed, the impact of enlightened and progressive human resources practices on performance (and in the private sector, profitability) has been widely acknowledged by a number of

The human resource in business planning

> **Box 5.1** Seven key areas of human resource practice to be addressed by managers
>
> 1. Review objectives, strategies and processes associated with people management
> 2. Monitor the satisfaction and commitment of employees on a regular basis
> 3. Monitor the culture of their organisations
> 4. Make organisational changes to promote job satisfaction and employee commitment
> 5. Review human resource management practices across the organisation
> 6. Receive training and support to provide vision and direction for the organisation's people management strategies
> 7. Ensure that the central element of the organisation's philosophy and mission is a commitment to the skill development, well being and effectiveness of all employees

leading management 'thinkers' in recent years (for example, Kanter 1985 and Harvey Jones 1992). More recently, a study of around 100 companies over a 7-year period (Patterson et al 1997) revealed that people management was one of the most critical factors in respect of business performance. The study highlights seven areas of human resource practice for managers to address (Box 5.1)

Similarly, Gratton (1997) reported the findings of her research into successful multinational companies which had identified that the human resources function in these organisations was central to their success. She advocates a 'systems model of people management' where human resources issues are not considered in isolation and where human resources professionals work alongside 'their line management business partners'. Such an approach requires managers at all levels to have an understanding of human resources issues and the important role they play in the delivery of the organisation's core business agenda. Effective human resource management is not the exclusive interest of human resource professionals but should be on the agenda of all those responsible for the management of other staff. It is therefore vital that all managers have an understanding of the role to be played by human resources in the wider business of the organisation. Good human resource practice has a direct impact on the staff of the NHS and ultimately influences the quality of care provided to patients.

Furthermore, it is essential that human resource professionals are firmly connected to the service delivery agenda of NHS

Delivering the business

organisations and do not restrict their role to that of the 'technical' expert. In consequence, human resources staff need to acquire a broader knowledge and skill base that acknowledges the wider contribution that they, as human resource professionals, can make to their organisation. For example, understanding the strategic role of human resource management, not only in its impact on service delivery but in the support of organisational change and development processes (knowledge about organisational design, culture, 'style' and communication become more important in this context). This requires the ability to work with and influence colleagues from a range of professional backgrounds (e.g. clinicians, accountants) and at a senior level within organisational management structures.

David Ulrich in his book, 'Human Resource Champions' (1997), has developed four metaphors to describe the role of the human resources professional: 'strategic partner', 'administrative expert', 'employee champion' and 'change agent'. In fulfilling these roles human resources professionals will need to possess not only the capacity to develop and use administrative infrastructures and be capable of handling a high level of continuous workforce change but most importantly will need to be strategic influencers. This will require them to work as effective enablers of change and internal change agents with the ability to think and act systemically, i.e. equipped to handle the complexity of structural, functional and workforce change and appreciate the necessary connections and interdependencies that have to be understood and managed. A connection with the core business of the organisation and an understanding of the concomitant development agenda will be vital.

Furthermore, if human resources professionals are to access available knowledge about best practice they will need to possess the skills to use and apply research. At its most basic this will require a level of 'research awareness', at its most sophisticated it may involve the human resources professional in gaining the skills to access funding to undertake and publish credible research which contributes to the evidence base of good human resource practice.

In summary, the human resources agenda cannot be divorced from the service agenda: how staff are organised, managed and developed has a direct impact on patient care and service development. The implication of this is that human resources issues should not be professionally bounded; they need to be of central concern to all managers throughout large, medium and small health organisations and across organisational boundaries.

151

The human resource in business planning

PART 2: WORKFORCE PLANNING (CAROL WILBY)

Workforce planning through the 1990s

Workforce planning has been carried out by the NHS in a variety of forms for many years. During the 1980s manpower planning activity utilised data from personnel files to determine the staffing requirements of each hospital and Health Authority. Individual staff groups were 'coded' according to the professional descriptors contained within the Whitley pay grades. In 1990, in an effort to improve supply and demand data for professional staff and link this to education and training requirements, and as part of a general review of the NHS, a UK government White Paper was produced, giving rise to the introduction of Working Paper 10 'Education and Training in the NHS' (WP10).

Working Paper 10 was the 10th White Paper to arise from the 1989 White Paper 'Working for Patients' (Department of Health 1989). It defined the responsibilities for non-medical health care professional preregistration education and training. The practice of contracting to support education purchasing was instigated in April 1991 by Regional Health Authorities (RHAs), mainly in response to the absence of accurate costing for educational provision. This contract activity was supported by workforce planning which projected and estimated the demand for NHS workforce requirements. The principles behind WP10 underlined the need for good supply and demand data in the form of robust workforce plans and the need to create a 'level playing field' in which education and training was seen as 'free at the point of delivery'.

April 1996 saw the abolition of the RHAs and the establishment of regional offices (ROs) in response to the Functions and Manpower Review (FMR) of the health service. As a consequence of this activity, and the subsequent downsizing of the NHS Executive, different arrangements needed to be developed to continue the commissioning of non-medical education and training (NMET). Alongside this management review of the NHS Executive came the integration of NHS colleges of health with higher education institutions (HEIs). This resulted in the need for a robust contracting framework to be developed in order to support the annual financial investment in non-medical health professional education and training of around £800 million.

In 1995 the NHS Executive introduced new policy arrangements to support the contracting framework through Executive

152

Letter EL(95)27 (Department of Health 1995). This EL announced new structures for the development and establishment of locally based education and training consortia, and suggested 'that the new arrangements would provide the health service with staff equipped with the knowledge and skills to be fit for the purpose of delivering health care'. The success of the NHS in meeting its objectives of promoting health, preventing disease and providing high-quality services and patient care is very much dependent upon achieving the right number of trained and motivated staff, able to meet the demands of the NHS into the twenty-first century. The membership of consortia was defined to reflect the changing patterns of health service commissioning and subsequent service delivery, and therefore includes representatives of Trusts, Health Authorities, social services, general practitioners (GPs) and private, voluntary and independent organisations.

For the first time, consortia bring together all health care employers to the same table, to debate the requirements for practice underpinned by education and training. One of the outcomes of this approach will be the creation of a dynamic link between education, training, employment and service delivery.

In England, 44 consortia were created as a result of this policy change. Their primary tasks are listed in Box 5.2.

Funding streams in support of non-medical education and training have also been subject to change, with the creation of a 'national' levy on Health Authorities being used to create the finances to support the commissioning of education. From 1 April 1998 this levy has supported two broad elements: (1) a core element mainly for pre-qualifying education and training required to enter a particular health care profession (determined by demand from service for new health care professionals and the cost of their training), and (2) a specialist and development element for education, training and the continuing development of the existing NHS health care workforce, where funding is both through the national levy and through financial investment by individual employers. (Greater understanding of the detail of

---

Box 5.2 Primary tasks for the education and training consortia

- To produce a workforce plan
- To commission education
- To monitor education contracts for quality, outcomes and return on investment
- To determine the strategic direction of education purchasing
- To advise on medical workforce requirements

The human resource in business planning

funding available and the staff groups to which it relates can be gained by reading the Health Service Circular (HSC) 1998/044 produced by the NHS Executive (Department of Health 1998b).)

Education and training consortia will be replaced by Workforce Development Confederations during 2001. These bodies will have the responsibility of ensuring the development of an appropriate workforce to meet the health needs of the population.

Workforce planning – the theory

It is clearly vital that workforce planning, as the driving force behind the estimation of staffing requirements, is dealt with in an appropriate manner and at the highest level in order to ensure the continued supply of well-educated, skilled and competent staff. Incremental changes to these processes are resulting in better intelligence regarding the state of the workforce and identification of potential difficulties in recruitment. For example current data suggest that the NHS is faced with an ageing workforce, and is set to lose 25% of its employees through retirement in the first 25 years of this century. This makes it imperative that we act now in order to ensure the continued supply of health care professionals.

Managers need to be able to forecast as robustly as possible their demands for qualified staff across the whole of the workforce planning time frame of 6 years. In order to achieve this managers must be encouraged to develop their workforce skills and ability as this will remain a high priority in the future. However, it is no wonder that managers have found it difficult to predict their requirements for staff when faced with service contracts being renewed on an annual basis, and when, for example, retirements are difficult to predict as they can occur over a 10-year time frame, and when recruitment is made difficult by previous decisions to reduce the level of education commissions placed. The move towards 3-year service agreements should make this a little easier, but other variables remain.

High-quality, robust workforce data can assist us in profiling the needs of the future workforce, and help overcome some of these inherent difficulties. The NHS currently holds data from 6 years of planning and is using this to analyse trends in retirements, ethnicity, age and recruitment profiles. This type of information will assist us in answering the questions: 'What type of skills will we require in 5 years time?' and 'How will we bridge the supply and demand gap?'

Delivering the business

In responding to these questions and to begin the process of workforce planning and profiling we must first ask more questions:

- Where is the organisation heading – what is its strategic direction?
- What are the core services?
- What are we to develop/withdraw from?
- What needs to be done to get us there – what is the focus of the annual business plan?
- What skills are needed to deliver the service – do they exist?
- If not, what is the gap?
- Who should do what?
- How do we apply the skills?
- How do we ensure skills develop the organisation and move it along?
- How do we plan today for the skills of the future?
- Will our plans meet our needs, or the needs of others?

Many of these questions relate to the organisation and its operating structures, so we must also ask questions of the resource underpinning its performance and success:

- Why do people leave?
- Where do we recruit staff from, and what makes them stay?
- How many of our staff are mature entrants and how many are returners to work?
- What is our turnover and wastage rate?
- How many of our staff work part time?
- What type of skill mix do we want?
- Is there a national skills shortage?

We must also remember that we are competing within the some labour market as our neighbours and therefore should understand who they are and their core business.

Changes to work-based and lifelong learning, the increasing use of occupational standards and changes to professional boundaries and practice will equally impact on the decisions we take in relation to the demand we originate through workforce planning for education and training commissions.

Workforce planning – the reality

The current cycle of workforce planning (Table 5.1) 'peaks' in early summer with the production of demand data by originated Trusts to support their business plans and the general strategic

The human resource in business planning

155

Table 5.1 Annual workforce planning cycle

Month	Workforce planning activity	Contracting/commissioning activity
March	Launch of workforce planning process	
April	Trusts commence data collection	Review meetings with higher education institutions re quality and outcomes
	Data requests to Health Authorities and social services	Strategic direction for services provided by Health Authorities
	Review of independent sector needs	
May		Ongoing contract performance management with higher education institutions
June	Trusts return data to consortia	
	Initial consortia plans to regional offices	
	Analysis back to Trusts	
July	Modification of plans	
Aug	Completed annual plan to regional offices	
Sep	Assessment of plan by regional offices/REDG	Commissioning plans approved by REDG
Oct	Financial assessment against NHS allocation from the levy	Indicative commissioning figures shared with higher education institutions
Nov		Ongoing contract monitoring
		Higher education institutions produce annual reports
		Formal approval for commissioning plans
		Letters of agreement/contracts produced
Dec		Final agreement of education costs
Jan		Ongoing contract performance management
Feb	Development of planning databases and guidance for the following year	
	Production of profiling data to assist in planning	

direction of service delivery and development. However, it must be noted that this is simply one phase in the year-long process and cannot be viewed in isolation, as the workforce planning cycle has equally important phases of financial determination and education contracting negotiations.

In many ways, the current process continues to ask the questions that were asked in the past, and therefore continues to perpetuate the 'planning in boxes' approaches of WP10, where the demand for each profession was viewed in isolation. However in response to this the questions asked are broadening to include all staffing data which may be relevant to the development of services and the commissioning of education.

It is equally important and therefore as valid to understand the skill mix changes underway within different organisations which are affecting the supply and demand of support staff. This approach becomes crucial in areas where skills shortages are occurring and recruitment is proving difficult. One of the most crucial questions to ask is: 'What is your demand for newly qualified staff?'. This is important when one considers that from the year of forecast to the year of being available to work as a qualified practitioner there is minimum time span of 4 years. That is to say that the nursing students requested today (2001), will not be available to recruit until 2005, year 1 in planning and 3 subsequent years of education. The data which feed this process are taken directly from the information returned by Trusts and other employing health care organisations; if the demand is not identified in this way, there will not be sufficient qualified staff in the 'pool' to recruit from. The key data flows and organisational relationships are depicted in Figure 5.1.

In moving towards a system of planning and data collection which allows us to picture or profile service areas and determine skills requirements across professional, vocational and academic boundaries we will be able to meet the ever changing needs of health care delivery. This integrated approach to workforce planning and profiling (as illustrated in Box 5.3) will ensure a cohesive, team response to delivering policy changes and result in effective, efficient delivery of both health services and health professional education, and move away from the 'planning in boxes' approaches of WP10.

In following this approach it is important to continue to ask similar questions to those detailed earlier, thereby enabling the consortia to ensure that workforce planning develops an understanding of the full range of future demands on the clinical workforce and uses this assessment to predict the shape of the whole workforce, linking across professional and employment boundaries, and education pathways. This process will enable assessment of the potential courses of action available for making the transition from the current shape of the workforce to a configuration for future delivery of health care focusing

The human resource in business planning

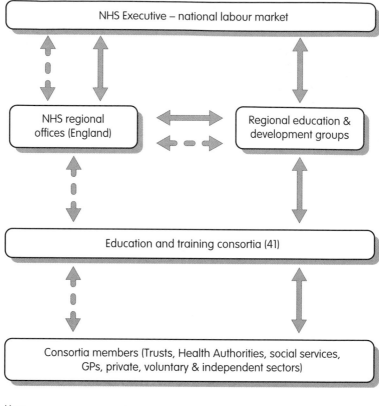

Figure 5.1 Organisational relationships and data flows.

on succession planning, skill mix reviews, recruitment and retention, continuing professional development and staff intention underpinned by an education strategy.

Workforce issues such as these can easily be seen as 'too difficult to handle'; however, high-quality, effective care can only be delivered to differing and diverse care groups if the right services and skills are available when required. In making decisions on the level of education commissions to be placed, the education consortium and ultimately the regional education and development group must take account of how their local workforce planning meshes with and informs the national picture to ensure 'the right skills, in the right place, at the right time'.

> **Box 5.3** An example of integrated planning: children's services
>
> - Determination of strategic direction of health care for children/paediatrics
> - Identification of local healthcare delivery/services (where, how, financial resource, partnerships)
> - Assessment and definition of skills required to deliver the service (competencies, standards and levels, not professional hierarchies)
> - Determination of types and numbers of professionals required (e.g. doctors, nurses, social workers, health visitors, school nurses, paediatric community nurses, psychologists, support staff, nursery places)
> - Assessment and determination of the number and type of education commissions to be placed

References

Audit Commission (1997) Finders, keepers: the management of staff turnover in NHS Trusts. London: The Stationery Office.

Department of Education and Employment (1998) The learning age – a renaissance for a new Britain. London: The Stationery Office.

Department of Education and Employment (1999) Learning to succeed – a new framework for post-16 learning. London: The Stationery Office.

Department of Health (1989) Working for Patients. London: HMSO.

Department of Health (1995) Commissioning non-medical education and training, EL(95)27. London: HMSO.

Department of Health (1997) The new NHS: modern, dependable. London: The Stationery Office.

Department of Health (1998a) Our healthier nation – a contract for health. London: The Stationery Office.

Department of Health (1998b) Funding non-medical education and training (HSC 1998/044). London: The Stationery Office.

Department of Health (1999) Saving lives: our healthier nation. London: The Stationery Office.

Gratton L (1997) Tomorrow people. People Management 24 July.

Handy C (1990) The age of unreason. London: Century Hutchinson.

Harvey-Jones Sir J (1992) Troubleshooter 2. London: BBC Books.

Kanter R (1985) The change masters: corporate entrepreneur at work. London: Allen & Unwin.

NHS Executive (1996) Creative career paths in the NHS – the agenda for action. London: Department of Health.

Patterson G M, West M A, Lawthom R, Nickell S (1997) Impact of people management practices on business performance. Issues in People Management No. 22. London: IPD.

Ulrich D (1997) Human resource champions. Boston, Massachusetts: Harvard Business School Press.

The human resource in business planning

Application 5:1 *Carol Wilby*

Workforce planning process

We have looked at the wider picture of human resource development and planning in Chapter 5. Here Carol Wilby provides a case study of a surgical directorate to demonstrate how the principles of workforce planning are applied. Try to make links with what you have read about the business planning activities in organisations, and think about the challenges of making plans in an environment of continual and continuous change.

The education and training of a workforce as vast and diverse as the NHS must have at its heart the culture and principle of good workforce planning. Because of its size and complexity we must ensure that we have a robust framework which underpins this ethos. This is why we create a division between pre- and post-registration activity, which is, in reality a continuous process of learning.

IN THE BEGINNING...

In order for us to understand our role in forecasting, educating and developing the workforce for the future we must first understand where we feature in the 'bigger picture'. Let us take the example of a staff nurse on a general surgical ward. Which part of the jigsaw of information do they hold? As the nurse already holds a professional pre-registration qualification you may ask yourself where they fit into the picture of demand assessment. However, it is precisely because of the qualification already held that we start here. All professional nursing staff must show evidence of continued education and development to remain on the United Kingdom Central Council (UKCC) register. This means that the majority of nurses will at some point in their career attend 'formal' education programmes, and will require release from their employer. Equally, employers will have their own perspective of the type of education required by staff in order for them to remain at the forefront of care delivery (i.e. fit for purpose in the workplace), and to ensure the delivery of service contracts and developments, as detailed in the organisation's business plan.

Understanding the pattern of release required, for example any time away from the ward, as well as the outcome (i.e. the qualification to be pursued), builds a picture of the amount of support needed by the individual in the form of mentoring, study leave, etc. The level of replacement (human resource) needed by the ward, and related costs, in order to maintain the service must be considered also.

APPRAISAL

Much of this information is gained through discussion during personal appraisal and objective setting and the subsequent development of a personal development plan (PDP). Through the use of this type of information the ward manager can build up a comprehensive picture of the needs of his or her staff in relation to education, training and development. This picture will be examined in the light of the current and future service needs. Within our surgical directorate, each ward manager will be carrying out this task, the results of which are then aggregated into the directorate's demand for post-registration education, training and development.

You can see from this example how important it is for each staff nurse to articulate his or her professional skills development needs, as this aggregated information will have a direct impact on the type of education and training commissioned through local education consortia.

THE THREE RS: RECRUITMENT, RETENTION AND RETIREMENT

Through the assessment and understanding of the turnover of staff within a directorate the manager can build a

Workforce planning process

picture of both recruitment and retention patterns. Recruitment data can tell us how easy or difficult it is to attract nurses with the appropriate skills and knowledge. These data will, of course, differ in areas of high demand specialisms; for example, we are struggling to attract intensive care nurses in some localities, whilst in other specialties, recruitment is not so difficult. Geography can influence these data too, as different areas have different recruitment patterns.

Recruitment data alone are not enough to build the picture of workforce demand, but must be used along with staff retention data, which show us the reason for the movement of staff to other organisations, and also gives the picture of movement between areas of practice within an organisation (staff 'churning'). Then we come to retirements! This is one of the most difficult areas to predict what might happen. Nurses can retire from the age of 55, and this is a matter of personal choice. Thus, we do need to build in 'educated guess' into our demand for staff, because of the length of time it takes to recruit and educate a replacement.

FISHING IN THE SAME POOL

So far, the collection of data has given us a picture of the workforce already in employment and its subsequent development needs. This information is crucial in helping us to determine if we are going to recruit staff from the wider workforce who are already experienced, or, are we looking to recruit the newly qualified practitioner straight from higher education.

Whichever way you choose to recruit, you must bear in mind that you are 'fishing from the same pool' as all other employers of nurses, and, in reality, most managers would look to achieve a balance between new and experienced staff. However, the most important note here is the demand for newly qualified nurses. The data captured through the process that we have been outlining are fed directly into the education commissioning process carried out by education consortia on an annual basis. Because of this, it is vitally important for managers to articulate the demand far enough in advance (1 year planning plus 3 years in training) for the nurses to be educated in time to meet the projected demand.

THE WIDER WORKFORCE

Having looked at the qualified workforce we must now turn our attention to the other staff who support them in carrying out the care given to patients on the surgical ward, as the nurses form only part of the staffing equation. The role and number of health care assistants along with their training needs must be taken into consideration, particularly when, in some instances, we are finding it difficult to recruit qualified staff.

The same consideration we gave earlier to appraisal and personal development plans must be given to support workers, including the ward clerical staff. It is only when we have done this that we can start to see the real picture of demand for human resources. Indeed this process must be followed for any member of staff who is part of the core team of the surgical ward. For example, in some cases, dedicated physiotherapy and occupation therapy services are attached to ward establishments.

THE FUTURE

We have come a long way in developing the processes of how we determine our need for staff. We have, however, still a long way to go until we can comfortably 'sit tight' and say we have got it right. In the future we must also be asking our medical colleagues the same questions in relation to numbers, skills and education; they are, after all, an integral and important part of care delivery. Integrating the process of workforce planning right across the board, including professions and organisations, is the only way to ensure that we meet as effectively as possible the staffing needs of the health and social care sector in the future.

Further reading

Department of Health (1998) Working together: securing a quality workforce for the NHS. London: The Stationery Office.

Workforce planning process

163

Personal development – a relationship between individual and organisation

Delivering the business

Personal development is a lifelong process. It occurs in the workplace, but also in our personal life. The person who develops in a proactive way has the flexibility of approach to be in touch with the fast changing world of work and society. This application focuses on the way in which the individual and the organisation can work together to achieve the best for both.

The language which is used when discussing employment suggests a great deal about how attitudes and priorities have changed. It seems not long ago when 'job description' was the key term. It created a picture of work delivered according to a set of templates. The organisation, having established the template, simply sought the employees to match the template. The idea was for the individual to fit the job description. The thought that he or she might contribute to, or enhance the scope of the job was hardly considered. It seemed that a job was a collection of tasks rather than an enterprise.

But now the word is 'contract'. Everyone – staff, full-time, part-time, freelance, interim, consultant – has a contract. It is the cornerstone of employment relationships and law. But the significance is much greater than the legal requirement.

Contract (Latin: *con*, together; *trahere*, to draw) means to 'draw together'. This is important in two ways. First, because it embraces the idea of the two-sided nature of the employment agreement. Secondly, and more crucially, because it advances the concept of two entities, the organisation and the individual, drawn together in a common purpose.

In the last decade every self-respecting organisation had a mission statement. While the pompous style of some of these was derided, and they are now displayed with more modesty, the ideas that fathered them have grown in strength. Successful organisations understand that their plans, objectives, aspirations and obligations need to be articulated in a corporate culture and value system.

So though the mission statement may have moved into the background, its components have increased in significance. As individuals we each have our own 'mission statement'. It may be unspoken, even subconscious, but ultimately it is what makes us tick.

A sound contract between organisation and individuals is one in which these two sets of ideas are drawn together so that they support each other. When this 'mutuality of aspiration' is recognized, when each side contributes to and is encouraged to be creative on behalf of the other, the automatic result should be growth for both. The ideal is that the process becomes organic. The Chinese proverb says: 'in the flourishing of each tree the orchard is fruitful'.

In what ways can we move towards this ideal? Certainly not by drawing apart in the workplace and in our development planning what we have drawn together in the process of organising employment (i.e. agreeing a contract).

When we join an organisation we bring to it a set of values, a personal identity and an individual potential, strongly shaped by our life experiences and the influences of others. But these shaping factors do not stop, so they prompt us to keep reviewing our attitudes and developing our management behaviours. The overall objective is to fulfil potential, be professional and flexible, and to demonstrate credible leadership, and to do this within a common framework of understanding. In parallel, the organisation has its 'mission statement' components, and these too evolve and develop.

The key words are 'in parallel'. Things are lost when the development lines diverge, either because one grows

Personal development

165

while the other stays still, or because both develop but towards different goals. So it is very important when you consider a job that you understand and share cultural values with the organisation. For success, affinity with the culture is more important than a first class honours degree.

Kouzes & Posner (1995) found in their research that individuals fall into three categories in relation to their value relationships with their organisations:

1. Those with great clarity about both personal and organisational values. These had the highest degree of commitment to the organisation.
2. Those with a clear view of their personal values but little awareness of the organisation's. These too had high commitment but below the first group.
3. Those without clarity about either their own or their organisation's values. This group had poor commitment and were most alienated from their work.

So it is apparent that clarity of personal vision is the first, essential step for success, on which must be built a clear vision about the organisation's own aims and principles. On this good ground both will have the best chance of success. Such ground is essential if deep roots are to be planted, and with the rising pace of change, only the trees with deep roots will be flexible enough to bend with the wind.

Unfortunately from the organisation's engine-room it is easy to lose sight of its strategic needs. I saw this demonstrated with a group of managers in a recent brainstorm to explore organisational needs. This group saw no common thread in what they were paid to achieve and the challenges facing the organisation. Almost worse, they did not feel in a position to influence how the business might respond to its challenges. They were not, in their view, empowered to do so.

Fortunately none of you need face such a depressing impasse. There are clear initiatives you can take. First is to review regularly your career plan. As the organisation's challenges and objectives will develop, your career plan should be flexible to dovetail with theirs. In order to respond to change, you need your own personal development plan. In some organisations this can be achieved through workshops and development centres provided by the organisation. Others depend on the appraisal system and performance reviews, possibly with employee/line manager dialogue and 360 degree feedback. But even if none of this is available there is nothing to prevent you working on your individual plan, on your own or with a trusted colleague or mentor.

THE TOOLS AVAILABLE

There are various tools you can use to work on your career plan or personal development plan.

The lifeline

Developed by Shepard & Hawley (1974) this exercise enables you to reveal the themes and patterns associated with high levels of motivation and fulfilment. First you draw your lifeline as a graph, with peaks a representing the highs of your past, valleys the lows. Go as far back as you can remember, at least to school days. You will get a feel for the comparative heights of the high spots in relation to one another. Note against each when the peak experience was, and why. What was going on in your life at that time? Then do the same for the valleys. With a highlighter colour the common characteristics in the peaks, then in the valleys. An experience creating a valley might be, for example, one of great frustration, at other times one that was painful. Frustration, though it makes you feel and behave badly, is actually an indicator of something significant in you, otherwise you would not invest emotional energy in it. So a frustration in a valley may be accentuating something which is a peak elsewhere in your graph.

The skill and knowledge audit

Ask yourself the following sequence of questions:

- What are the aims of the organisation?
- What am I paid to achieve?

Personal development

- What do I do well?
- What do I do less well?
- What actions do I need to take to address the things I do less well?

Write your answers on small self-stick notes, one per note, and as many as possible per question. Now colour code the answers. Where an answer conveys something the organisation values highly, put a small green sticker or dot on it, where it refers to something you enjoy, put a gold/yellow sticker or dot and where it identifies something you know you need to do better, use the colour red. The resulting colour groupings will help you to identify where the emphasis of your personal development plan should be placed.

Imagery

The use of metaphor and analogy can be very valuable in creating a vision of your future. Imagine, for example, your ideal form of transport, with all the features your heart can desire. Maybe it is a fantasy machine, maybe something more realistic. Sketch it, using plenty of colour, no inhibition. Play with the image. Now, look at it for a few minutes, then note by the drawing the qualities and characteristics of this form of transport.

Next, do the same exercise again, but this time draw the mode of transport to represent your here-and-now. (If my current life were a form of transport, what would it look like?) Again when you finish, capture the ideas in words beside the image.

It would be unhelpful in this exercise to think in terms of positives and negatives. We all make hard decisions and trade-offs, work versus family for example. These are, however, calculated choices. The real problems are more commonly linked with lack of control over our lives.

Every now and then re-visit your here-and-now image. See if there are any adaptations you could make to it to improve it, to give it some of the features of the ideal. When working with images it is important to think what the features mean for you. Power, for example, is for some people negative, for others exciting. Speed may be positive and attractive to some, intimidating and dangerous to others. Avoid being judgemental. What is a strength in one role or corporate culture may be a weakness in another.

These are some suggestions for do-it-yourself analysis to help in your personal development planning. There are many others, but whichever you use, the ingredients that ultimately will inform your development plan are:

- Your skills
- Your motivation
- Your experience
- Your specialist knowledge
- Your beliefs
- Your potential for development
- Your appreciation of the organisation's needs
- Your understanding of the nature of the partnership between you.

THE PRACTICAL FEATURES OF YOUR PERSONAL DEVELOPMENT PLAN

The intention in the NHS was that the majority of employees would have a personal development plan by April 2000. You should think through for yourself:

1. the competency areas you want to work on and how these dovetail with the organisation's needs,
2. your current operating level of competency,
3. the level you want to reach in line with the organisation's change and growth objectives,
4. your planned learning activities, which may include training but rarely training courses exclusively, and
5. ideas on how your behaviour/performance will be changed by the plan. This would include proposals for measurement of development achieved or examples of new skill or knowledge in practice.

None of this is as intimidating as it may appear at first glance. You can think them through informally, and if possible discuss them with a trusted friend or colleague, or your mentor. It can form the basis for your review or appraisal with your manager.

Take ownership of your own development – you are worth the investment!

Personal development

169

References

Kouzes J, Posner B (1995) The leadership challenge. San Francisco: Jossey-Bass.

Shepard H A, Hawley J A (1974) Life planning and organisations. Washington DC: National Training and Development Services Press.

Delivering the business

Chapter **Six**

The business of finance

Con Egan

- **Financial pressures**
  National funding
- **Distribution of funds within the health system**
- **Internal financial control – an explanation**
  Costs

- **The importance of planning**
- **References**

OVERVIEW

Financial activity has always been present in the NHS but its profile increased enormously following the introduction of the internal market. Despite current softening of the competitive ethos, financial and resource management are here to stay, and it is important that all staff in health care provision understand how finance is managed. It is fair to say that many clinical professionals are uncomfortable with the notion of having to consider cost when caring for patients. However, this is a reality of life which is with us permanently, and Con Egan presents a brief overview of financial issues in the NHS in a straightforward and readable way. Remember that the combined expertise of both financial and clinical professionals is more likely to achieve the best outcome for the patient.

When describing the financial management of health care it is useful to focus on three particular areas to gain clarity:

1. Helping people to gain a better understanding of where the money for the NHS comes from and how it flows through the system.
2. Describing how resources are managed by clearing away the jargon to help to gain a better understanding of some of the terms used by accountants. The principles, in fact, are quite simple but it takes the genius of an accountant to make them sound complex!
3. Exploring the extent to which finance can help an organisation to think through what its priorities are within the parameters of a limited budget.

FINANCIAL PRESSURES

National funding

To return to the first issue – where does the money come from? Some myths need to be dispelled. The NHS is not funded out of the 'NHS stamp' nor from our insurance contributions, any more than the roads programme is funded out of the road tax. The government acquires income from a variety of sources, primarily income tax, value added tax and corporation tax. It then spends the money on a variety of services. The government is very reluctant to have particular income raised for specific purposes. To an extent this takes away the government's prime role in determining priorities between expenditure. At a recent general election – not for the first time – one of the parties came forward with the proposal to have a particular amount of income tax raised to be spent on health and/or education. Any such tax would be technically termed a hypothecated tax, but in the British government systems there are very few examples of this having been sustained.

Essentially, there are almost two separate processes, although with clear overlaps: the government acquires income through taxation and the government determines expenditure. Until a few years ago these two processes appeared, at least to the person in the street, to be completely separate. Most of us will remember the annual budget in late

Delivering the business

March/early April which seems to determine from where the government will raise income. Despite being called a budget, it in no way spells out where the money will be spent. By the time the budget is announced (a few days before, or in fact just after, the commencement of the financial year) the decision on expenditure has long since been made.

At this point it is perhaps worth pointing out that in Britain the tax year runs from 6 April through to the following 5 April, whilst government financial years are from 1 April to the following 31 March. These strange dates for the tax year stem originally from the financial year beginning on Lady Day, the first quarter day in the year – 25 March. When Britain 'lost' 11 days in changing onto the Gregorian calendar in 1752, the taxman still insisted on his 11 days! Ever since then the year end has been 5 April.

Whilst in one sense this might seem to be totally irrelevant, it does reflect the extent to which the whole funding system in Britain is very much determined by our history. This is most obvious in the continuing splitting of the receipt of income by government and the insistence of Parliament on voting money to government on an annual basis. This goes back to the English Civil War and the insistence by Parliament at the restoration of the monarchy in 1660 that it would vote money to the monarchy only on an annual basis, i.e. it would determine the level of money the government would be allowed to expend. Nowadays it might seem that government determines the amount of money and Parliament facilitates the process rather than the other way round, but legally Parliament still has the right to vet and vote for that money annually.

Government clearly focuses most of its attention on the level of expenditure and the balance of priorities. As we have already said, until recently the annual budget focused on income but now there is a much clearer, much closer interface between the two processes. Decisions on what will be spent in any particular year are finally made in the autumn of the previous year. This follows a long process of formal and informal negotiations involving the Treasury and individual Departments of State to agree the expenditure that they will be expected to manage within the following period.

The key players in all this process are the prime minister (the prime minister is First Lord of the Treasury) and chancellor of the exchequer. They will begin the process by identifying the total amount of public expenditure for the year and the policy framework within which decisions will be made.

You will not be surprised to find that the target amount for total public expenditure is always less than individual departments feel they need for their services. The reference to 'formal and informal' alludes to the fact that whilst there are official Whitehall processes, where a group of senior ministers clearly take the lead in reviewing the potential level of expenditure in future years, one cannot underestimate the part played by informal lobbying, leaks to the press, etc. The end product of all these debates is decisions endorsed by Cabinet in late autumn about the level of public expenditure to be met and the amount allocated to each department. Table 6.1 shows a recent analysis of public expenditure. The first thing to notice is the vast extent of public expenditure. Tables always tend to focus on billions of pounds rather than just millions or mere thousands. This tells its own tale. A figure that might surprise is the extent of expenditure coming under the auspices of social security. Without

Table 6.1 1998/99 national budget (all figures shown in billions)

Expenditure		Income	
Social security (includes cyclical social security)	£ 96.6	Income tax	£ 84.3
Welfare to work	£ 1.1	Corporation tax	£ 30.0
Health	£ 37.2	VAT	£ 53.3
Local government	£ 32.7	Petrol duty	£ 21.5
Scotland, Wales, N. Ireland	£ 29.9	Tobacco duty	£ 8.9
Defence	£ 22.2	Drink duties & gambling	£ 8.3
Employment & education	£ 13.0	Business rates	£ 15.0
Home Office	£ 6.9	Social security contributions	£ 53.7
Transport	£ 12.1	Council tax	£ 11.6
Local authority (self-financed expenditure)	£ 14.0	Interest & dividends	£ 4.5
Reserve	£ 3.0	Windfall tax	£ 2.6
Debt interest	£ 24.6	Other	£ 36.5
Other spending	£ 39.2		
		Total income	£ 330.2
		Public sector borrowing requirement	£ 2.3
Total expenditure	£ 332.5		£ 332.5

opening the debate here, when one thinks of the likely age profile of the UK population over the next 30 or 40 years, the financial challenge facing government can be seen. Expenditure in this area is difficult to curtail and, of course, the income side is going to be drawn from a smaller proportion of the population. More people will be beyond retirement age and therefore not contributing as much to the national coffers.

The challenge for government will continue, therefore, to be to try to balance the income and expenditure as appropriate. It is fair to say, however, that it is very rare that a government actually wishes to have a complete balance in any one particular year. Public expenditure deficits are not necessarily a 'bad thing'. Public expenditure is, after all, only one part of the totality of a country's economy. When the private sector is struggling there are strong arguments for an expansion in the public sector to maintain an equilibrium in the total economy. Economics is not just about planning expenditure but is primarily about creating an environment in which people have meaningful work and where the totality of developments for a population is maximised.

Throughout the twentieth century most large western economies have spent more years with a deficit than a surplus. It can be argued that this is actually creating a larger burden for future generations because essentially deficits are funded out of borrowing, but there is a need for balance in this area. One would not want to see a deficit becoming so all-consuming that the payment of interest becomes too large a burden, but there is a very strong case to be made that investment in infrastructure, be it transport, education or health, can be reasonably funded out of borrowing because the benefits gained in the future will be paid for by future generations. Most people, after all, fund their own major long-term investment (housing) out of borrowings.

DISTRIBUTION OF FUNDS WITHIN THE HEALTH SYSTEM

We need to move on now from the actual decision making at national level to how the funds are then distributed within the health service, describing the layers at which allocations are handled and what methodologies are used to determine the actual size of allocations.

At all levels of health service there are two dimensions of expenditure from Cabinet determination right down to the

The business of finance

smallest department within the service. All managers, whilst arguing for more resource for their service, are trying to contain expenditure within their area and perhaps, as part of this, controlling disbursement down to a lower level. The secretary of state for health argues for more money for health and then becomes the arbitor as to how that money will be spent within various parts of the health sector, social services, etc. Once that money has been allocated down to Health Authority level the Health Authority itself goes through the same process. Trusts themselves then go through that same process internally, considering how this money should be spent within their own departments, and departmental heads will go through the same process and argue for how the resource is to be managed. There is, therefore, an expectation that in controlling expenditure people will also be conscious of the need to 'argue their corner'.

To return now to the national picture. The system has changed a number of times during the last 50 years. For almost all that time (up to 31 March 1996) most of the money from the department was fed through Regional Health Authorities (RHAs), previously Regional Health Boards (RHBs). These would cover areas with populations broadly of 3–4 million people and covering areas such as the West Midlands and the North West. The number of regions was rationalised from 14 to eight in 1994, thus creating regions that covered a large area of population.

Before 1994 each region determined how to allocate resources to each of its constituent districts below that. The next level down was usually focused around a city or town, usually called a district. Since Regional Health Authorities were abolished the allocations have actually gone direct from the department to district level.

The debate about ensuring allocations were as fair as possible only really began in the 1970s. For the first 25 years of the NHS allocations were essentially incremental based on 'last year plus a bit'. The only significant change in allocations would follow the opening of a new significant development (usually a new hospital) where there would be recognition of the extra revenue requirements. The technical phrase used then and now was the revenue consequence of capital schemes (RCCS for short). Strategic shifts in resources were therefore very much capital/development led. A number of points arise from this:

● Except where there had been major capital developments, the inequities in distribution of health resources when the NHS was established in 1948 still prevailed.

Delivering the business

- The basis of deciding what new developments would go ahead was as likely to be political as on any assessment of greatest need. 'Political' in this sense would be at least as much to do with influence as with party politics, and may be completely the opposite to the assessment based on need. After all, health facilities prior to 1948 were better established where there were powerful interests – universities, major benefactors, etc. These influences could still be there.
- In the way developments were approved (even if they had been strategically targeted on the basis of need and no financial discipline was imposed) 'the bigger the better' was the order of the day. Imagine a system where houses were allocated freely on this basis. How many people would settle for a small, end-terraced house? We will come back to this later when we discuss capital charges.

Two factors came together in the mid-1970s to change this picture. First, there was a government determined to do something to bring about a greater sense of fairness, but secondly and, perhaps far more importantly, it became possible to see more clearly the range of differences in allocation per head. This was a result of the significant changes in health service structure brought about in 1974. Prior to that, hospital services funds primarily were administered via a very large number of hospital management committees. Mental health services, for example, were mainly provided through large psychiatric institutions providing services for large populations crossing many local authority boundaries, as there was no easy way to match these hospitals to particular populations. Furthermore, many of the new community services had previously been funded through local authorities. The 1974 reorganisation created Area Health Authorities, co-terminous with revised (and larger) local authorities. It was, therefore, a relatively simple process to compare area allocation with specific population.

This comparison was too crude a measure for a number of technical reasons discussed later. In the days before the introduction of the internal market, it was not accounted for that some areas (particularly teaching districts) provided significant services to people outside their boundaries, and thus there was still an obvious mismatch of resources. The oft-quoted example is that the spend per head was twice as much in some parts of the south of England as in Leicestershire. This mismatch led to the establishment of a Resource Allocation Working Party (RAWP), which began work on determining a methodology for establishing 'fair shares'. Whilst this work continues (and the debate will probably be never ending) there is little doubt that this process has shaved the extremes and brought a much greater sense of fairness to resource allocations.

Whilst the prime determinant of an allocation at any district (previously region) was the population, the actual allocation would never be based precisely on its population for a number of reasons. The first and most important reason is that the starting point in determining an allocation is what any particular organisation received in the previous year. The main reason for this has always been a desire to handle change sensitively and not to create major upheaval in any particular service. If one part of the country is receiving 20% more than another, clearly this is undesirable, but if it were adjusted all at once there would be major issues in relation to staff numbers and closure of facilities in one area and an inability to recruit and spend the money in developing facilities in another.

Another major reason why allocations have not been exactly equal to population is that population itself is too crude a measure. People of different ages use the health services to a greater or lesser extent. People up to the age of 15 and those over the age of 65 use the health service most, and in the middle 50 years use is much lower. Thus it is necessary to divide the population into relevant age groups. Again, self-evidently, use between the age of 0 and 5 is higher than between 5 and 15, and at the other end of the age spectrum use by people over the age of 75 is more than by those between 65 and 75. Using this information a weighted population profile, i.e. a population profile weighted according to age group, is achieved.

The actual weightings are based on evidence of patient use and actual costs incurred by different age groups. Putting it simply, this allows for the fact that a population formed mainly of very young children and elderly people will use more health resources than an area with a normal share of population. This is quite an issue in those areas where large numbers of elderly people congregate, e.g. coastal towns, and where a higher proportion of young children reside, new towns being obvious examples.

Basing the formula on aggregated weighted population would be sufficient if there were no factors other than age which affected people's need for services. The fact that other demographic factors have an impact on the differing needs for health has been acknowledged for a long time. This has become more explicit in the Green Paper 'Our Healthier Nation' (Department of Health 1998) and the subsequent White Paper, 'Saving Lives: Our Healthier Nation' (Department of Health 1999) which confirm the comments made in earlier documents such as the Black Report (Department of Health and Social Security 1980), which highlighted the impact on health needs of such factors as unemployment and poverty. Poverty and deprivation add to the likelihood of ill health so this is now taken into account in calculating 'fair shares'.

It is a challenge to identify the most accurate measures of need. Anecdotally, various suggestions are made, such as unemployment, but the key task is to establish a robust relationship between data on demographic factors that is easily available and their impact on health care. Working towards this, a significant amount of work was done during the 1990s, using highly sophisticated statistical techniques to arrive at a number of key factors which reflect need. One of the key factors was the robustness of the data collection process. The use of census data, for example, was often seen as advantageous because the data were being collected routinely, and in most cases have a high level of accuracy and credibility.

It is important to emphasise that this exercise is as much of an art as a science. There are debates still continuing as to the right choice of factors. People in country areas, for example, continually argue that dispersed provision adds to expense and should be considered. At present there is little clear evidence of this but this does not stop the debate. Similarly, there are arguments about the influence of ethnic backgrounds, but to what extent, for example, do these factors also show up in the unemployment problem and how do you avoid double-count?

In the context of this chapter we can only acknowledge that this debate continues. People who have a particular interest can read further, as much has been written which addresses not only on the current basis of the formula but on how this formula might be used at discrete levels. This becomes more of an issue following the recent White Paper 'The New NHS: Modern, Dependable' (Department of Health 1997) as allocations are likely to be based closer to individual practices within Primary Care Groups.

Recognising that the calculation of the formula is not a precise science, it seems that the imprecisions matter less as the figures become larger because there is less tendency for one particular feature to distort the overall pattern. There is, for example, still an element of the formula which is based on the standard mortality rate for an area. Standard mortality rate

The business of finance

essentially examines the number of deaths in an area against the number expected for that population and is obviously affected by the number of premature deaths. One can appreciate that in an area with a population of a million, two or three extra deaths in a period because of an unfortunate accident will have minimal effect on the figures despite the impact at a very local level of those deaths.

The use of standard mortality rates as a measure of need has always been contentious because in a sense it measures early death, not continuing morbidity, and there are arguments as to the extent to which early death follows morbidity. Clearly, it does if it is the result of a chronic illness but not all early deaths are brought about by this. This in itself leads into the old argument which revolved around 'targeting' resources. To target resources on areas of higher death rates clearly makes sense in order to tackle problems but does not act as a strong motivating factor. Improved health reduces funding!

The White Paper 'The New NHS: Modern, Dependable' (Department of Health 1997) focuses on the future of the NHS very much from a primary care perspective, and while this is to be welcomed it does certainly present challenges in allocating resources, particularly in establishing reliable data at such discrete levels. Much of the data on which demography is based stem from census returns or other data established at a local authority level. Even for that data capable of being broken down to individual enumeration districts or even postcodes – and not all are – there are difficulties at practice level. The fundamental difficulty is that it is very rare, particularly in cities, for any medical practice to be totally self-contained within a particular area. There is a lot of geographical crossover between practices. This leads to a practice having patients from a large number of enumeration districts. More important, this leads to a situation where most enumeration districts have patients from a variety of practices.

In allocating resources at practice level based on demographic information one is forced to begin to make assumptions, e.g. that the individual practices have a similar make-up of clients. Actual experience suggests that this is not true and that differing practices tend to attract different clients.

One of the attractive aspects of the establishment of Primary Care Groups and Trusts is that at this level (i.e. population circa 100 000) it is much easier to come to views about levels of need. Any distortions caused by one-off events have less impact. Thus, it is easier to establish 'fair shares' at a Primary Care

Group/Trust level. One can only counsel extreme caution in trying to go beyond.

This, of course, does create a dilemma for the new organisations which are being established. Consider this scenario. If the Primary Care Trust/Group is overspending it will want to establish exactly where that overspend lies and thus will need to look at individual practices. Great care must be taken in the way the practice share of an overall budget is interpreted. If, for example, because of its style one practice attracts a significant number of drug users, it will need more than a 'fair share'. How is this going to be defined and established?

This issue must be dealt with very carefully if the entire process of developing Primary Care Groups is not to suffer a severe loss of credibility. Nevertheless the search for greater levels of equity of access to funds at more discrete local levels must be encouraged. If reasonable levels of equity have been achieved at the district level, there is considerable evidence that there are marked inequities at more local levels. Proximity to facilities and/or the ability to influence local decision making seem to have significant impact on the level of service locally.

INTERNAL FINANCIAL CONTROL – AN EXPLANATION

In describing some key features of internal financial control in a jargon-free way, it is important to clarify some of the common words and phrases. Financial expenditure is referred to as either 'capital' or 'revenue'. At its simplest, capital is expenditure on any item which has a life of more than 12 months. Revenue is expenditure on items that continually recur. The word revenue, comes from the French *revenir* – 'to come again, to recur'. In that sense revenue expenditure is recurring, regular expenditure, and the most obvious example of that would be wages.

There are many potential debates and nuances in defining expenditure. It could be argued, somewhat facetiously, that the purchase of a can of beans with a life of 18 months could be described as 'capital'. This, of course, would be regarded as inappropriate and so what has evolved over the years has been a categorisation of capital as needing to satisfy two criteria: first, as already said, the item of purchase must have a life of well over a year; and second, the minimum level of expenditure is a key criterion. One difficulty with this second criterion is that different organisations identify different amounts of money to define that and, of course, over the year these amounts change. One illustration of this is that whilst the definitions of 'capital' will always be consistent within the health service they will differ from the definitions used in local authorities. In broad terms, large expenditure on long-term products with a long life is defined as capital.

Why does it matter whether an item is revenue or capital? In a sense this goes back to an earlier part of the chapter where we referred to annual expenditure and annual borrowing. It is a common experience to regard a long-term investment differently from a recurrent commitment. Borrowing for a house is felt to be more legitimate because you can pay for it over the length of the period of benefit. This is regarded as much more legitimate than borrowing for day-to-day expenditure. Borrowing money on a Wednesday to pay for bread and milk does lead to problems in the longer term. At a macro-economic level, it is therefore important to differentiate between expenditure to invest in the future and expenditure that essentially 'keeps the ship afloat'.

In the NHS up until recently capital was unfortunately a 'free gift' in a sense that there was no acknowledgement of the requirement to pay it back over the period of benefit. Major developments in service were delivered through the establishment of capital facilities – new hospitals particularly – and whilst strategically this helped to develop services, there was no financial discipline in the process. If a local area was successful in acquiring approval for a new hospital it also received the money to run it. Necessary – but not very disciplined.

Since the introduction of capital charges at the beginning of the 1990s this has changed. Capital charges recognise two aspects of any major capital purchase. First, the need to repay money borrowed to fund the development (and the need to spread this repayment over the time of benefit). Second, the need to begin developing a means of funding future purchases whilst recognising that the value of the asset itself is diminishing and depreciating.

The first element in essence is now taken account of by the fact that Trusts pay interest on debts. When Trusts were first established, the extent of borrowing matched the value of their assets. Half their assets were funded out of interest-bearing debt, the other half out of public dividend capital – the equivalent of shares in most companies. As a Trust continues to repay interest on debt for the assets they have, it also needs to account for the loss in value of these assets. The technical term for this is 'depreciation'. Capital charges cover both these items. Depreciation is calculated on an estimated life basis and these estimated levels are standard for differing items. For example, computers are depreciated over 5 years and hospitals usually up to 60 years.

In any one year, of course, new capital expenditure will not exactly match the amount by which current assets are depreciated. If you can envisage two neighbouring district general hospitals, one (Trust A) 90 years old, the other (Trust B) brand new. Trust A will almost certainly require more capital expenditure on refurbishment etc. than Trust B, but will be depreciating less (it is rather similar with cars). Trust A will be expecting a far greater capital allocation than will be garnered purely from the depreciation collected in capital charges. Trust B will have less expectation (even if not abandoning hope). Assuming that both Trusts broke even in terms of revenue income and expenditure, their differing requirements for cash to fund their capital programmes would be reflected in very different external financing limits (EFLs). Essentially, this is the power given to Trusts to borrow cash. If contract income matches revenue expenditure, then Trust A will need to borrow extra cash to fund the gap between the size of the capital programme and its depreciation income. It will require a positive EFL. Trust B is likely to be expected to repay cash – the excess depreciation charge – and will have a negative EFL.

One final thought on this: it could be said that the national amount of increase in EFL in any one year would reflect the extent to which the health services, capital stock had improved, i.e. the amount by which new capital exceeded the amount of lost value. Recognising, however, the extent to which the methods used to calculate depreciation are somewhat arbitrary, one should treat any such interpretation with great care.

An added dimension over the last few years has been the extent to which capital schemes have been funded via the private finance initiative (PFI) mechanism rather than directly from government funding. There are, of course, differing views on the relative benefits of PFI, but it is now very clear that involvement of and partnership with the private sector is here to stay. The perceived advantages include:

● The potential to increase the totality of funding available. The private sector is not as constrained as the public sector over the totality of funding. If a scheme makes good commercial sense then money can usually be found. Alas

The business of finance

this has not been the history of the public sector, where somewhat arbitrary limits have been imposed in the interest of governmental macro-economic policy (particularly the extent of public sector borrowing).

- The opportunity to bring into the service commercial rigours, discipline and enterprise. Some of the aspirational capital schemes developed in the past would be very unlikely to survive the rigours of a commercial review.
- Perhaps most crucially (although much less transparent) PFI gave the government the opportunity to put more funds into the revenue stream. In very difficult years for public sector funding this transfer from public sector capital to revenue certainly helped to alleviate the potential adverse impact of tight financial settlements for the Department of Health.

However, as far as the first point is concerned, this could of course work to the disadvantage of the health sector. The price of borrowing (interest rates), like most prices, is essentially determined by the balance between supply and demand. When funds are in short supply in the overall economy, the price will increase, and there is theoretically no guarantee that any health capital schemes would be funded.

Whilst the final point discussed above may have had short-term political value, it may not have been in the long-term interest of the service. Nevertheless, there is little doubt that the second advantage – increased rigour – has to be welcomed as the lack of discipline in the allocation of NHS capital cannot be defended. The oft-quoted question 'would you invest in this if it was your own money?' is now truly brought into focus.

Moving from capital to revenue, we will now focus on how Trusts receive income and what is meant by their 'three financial targets'. As discussed earlier, Health Authorities currently receive their funds based, at least broadly, on their population. This recognises that their responsibility is to ensure the delivery of services appropriate for their local populations. The actual services are provided almost entirely by NHS Trusts who are responsible for the provision of whatever services Health Authorities determine are necessary. Trusts – particularly large Teaching Hospital Trusts – are likely to provide services for patients from more than one local area, and are funded by the appropriate Health Authorities. For example, a large provincial teaching hospital will provide services to a number of neighbouring Health Authorities and will have been paid for this provision by means of a variety of contractual arrangements

Delivering the business

prior to the implementation of the 1997 White Paper 'The New NHS: Modern, Dependable' (Department of Health 1997).

These contracts might have been based on a particular charge per episode of care and usually described as a 'cost per case' contract. Alternatively, the contract might have been based on a level of payment to deliver a total service, usually for a period of one year. This is usually described as a 'block contract'. Contracts have an element of cost based on the establishment of the infrastructure required whatever the level of service delivered, and partly on the amount of cost determined by the level of throughput. This recognises that some element of cost (particularly around the use of buildings, heating, etc. but also some minimum level of staffing) is fixed at least in the short term, but that some costs are marginal. The costs vary depending on the actual throughput. Good examples of such costs might include drugs, food, etc. Such contracts are usually referred to as 'fixed and variable contracts'.

It was the introduction of the internal market which resulted in formalised contracts between the purchasers and providers of care. The publication of 'The New NHS: Modern, Dependable' and its sister papers heralded a change in the arrangements: contracting was believed to develop an adversarial relationship between purchasers and providers and also required a great deal of administrative input to let the contracts on a yearly basis. As a result of the abolition of the internal market brought about by the Health Act (1999) the new NHS is moving towards collaboration and partnership arrangements and whilst the split is still apparent, the arrangements have softened a little. Contracts are giving way to 'service agreements' and these are usually agreed for a period of at least 3 years. Not only are administrative costs reduced, but the longer term agreements encourage investment in the service which would be untenable if the contract had a life of only one year.

Costs

It must be appreciated that in the long term at least, no cost is fixed for ever. Even buildings can be closed, and staff contracts completed or terminated. Furthermore, movement in costs relating to increases in throughput, referred to as 'marginal costs', rarely conform to a nice straight line progression. After a time there are other savings brought about by bulk buying, greater efficiency, etc., or there may be the need to increase staffing or

The business of finance

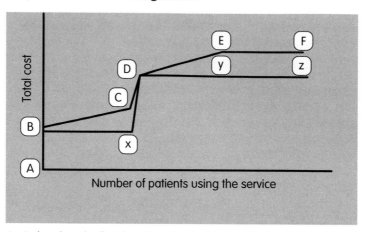

A→B descibes the **fixed cost** required whatever the level of service
B→C describes the **variable cost** of x patients
C→D describes the **stepped cost** required once x patients are exceeded
D→E describes the **variable cost** for y – x patients
E→F describes the lower variable cost of z – y patients brought about
through greater efficiency/purchasing power or whatever

Figure 6.1 Stepped costs.

building capacity beyond a certain level of demand. The latter changes in cost are usually termed 'stepped costs' (Fig. 6.1).

The contracts described earlier are an attempt to reflect the different cost drivers. These contracts essentially are the means by which Trusts receive their income. There will, of course, be occasions when patients from perhaps more distant Health Authorities are treated. This is usually as the result of an accident, and these are currently referred to as 'extra contractual referrals' (ECRs) and are charged simply at the expected average cost per case for the particular area of treatment. It is true to say that this area of the 1990 reforms has been particularly contentious, not least because of the significant amount of bureacracy involved in chasing relatively small amounts of income. The Labour government scrapped the system from 1 April 1999, and the replacement mechanism is not yet mature. Whilst for most organisations it can clearly be said that the amount of effort did not justify the result, there are, of course, particular issues for providers of services situated where there are large numbers of short-term visitors of very specialist services, particularly in coastal resorts and London.

Trusts, therefore, receive income almost entirely via contract, and their first, and perhaps most crucial financial duty is to

Delivering the business

ensure that their expenditure does not exceed this income. They must, in technical terms, break even, i.e. ensure that the two match. A Trust's second financial duty relates to what we said earlier about their external financial limit (EFL). Essentially, this relates to the amount of cash they require, assuming they break even, to balance their approved capital programme, taking account of that amount of capital charges they receive to fund the programme. Whilst technically this is their borrowing limit, to all intents and purposes this means the amount of cash they require from the Department or indeed intend to repay to the Department. As usual, life is rarely as simple as that. There will, for example, be recognition of the fact that Trusts are expected to earn income on their cash flow. The key point is that this EFL is agreed with the Department and must be adhered to.

A Trust's third target also relates to the value of their assets. Essentially, a Trust like any other organisation is expected to make best use of its capital assets, and they are expected to achieve an agreed 'rate of return' on these assets. This is usually expressed as a percentage. This will be primarily achieved by the receipt of that element of capital charges relating to the repayment of interest on the borrowings that funded the capital investment initially. There is a clear incentive for Trusts to maximise the use of those assets, so gaining more money, or to dispose of them, so reducing their interest commitment. This is yet another example of the extent to which the 1990 reforms began to put a long overdue emphasis on the use of expensive fixed assets.

Thus, the best way to maximise efficiency in costs is usually to look at the use of so-called 'fixed assets'. The element of efficiency gained through greater purchasing power or other efficiencies is usually relatively marginal compared to that potentially gained through rigorous appraisal of the use of capital stock.

When Trusts were first introduced, the first wave in 1991, the three statutory responsibilities, to break even, to stay within external financing limits (EFLs) of the organisation and to make 6% return on capital, were managed on a single year-by-year basis. As the changes in financial management roll out in the new NHS (i.e. post White Papers) NHS Trusts have one key financial obligation, that is to break even on an income and expenditure basis taking one year with another. This gives Trusts some flexibility in that they may, in certain circumstances, negotiate with a regional office to recover a poor financial position in subsequent years, normally up to 3 years.

The business of finance

In the same vein, Health Authorities have a statutory obligation not to go over their approved cash limit allocations, although they are allowed, but not encouraged, to carry forward a small (limited to 0.25%) planned underspend, whereas initially, books had to be closed at the end of the financial year.

THE IMPORTANCE OF PLANNING

> The great thing is not so much where we are, but in what
> direction we are going.
>
> Oliver Wendell Holmes

This section explores how an organisation's clarity of thinking around priorities and achievable objectives can be facilitated through the budgetary process, as it is crucial to see this process within the overall context of managing the agenda of an organisation.

Like many of the words and phrases used in describing financial management, the word 'budget' itself has many definitions. The following definition essentially encapsulates the theme of this section; it describes a budget as: 'A plan defining an organisation's key objectives and the various resources it intends to use to deliver these objectives'.

One concern that has emerged is that the very process of budgetary control, with its necessary emphasis on the provision of timely, relevant and detailed information to enable prompt and appropriate action to be taken, can lead to overemphasis on the short-term detail. The most important feature of a budget is the opportunity it gives an organisation to develop a plan to deliver its objectives. The process of identifying the appropriate resources should be the secondary process.

It could be argued that over the last 20 years in the public sector, the pressure on financial resources had totally dominated the agenda. This has often led to short-term measures to cope with 'crises' rather than an emphasis on long-term strategies. On the other hand, certainly in the late 1990s, the recognition that financial pressures in the public sector are here to stay has begun to encourage key questions such as:

- What is our purpose?
- Where do we best add value?
- Where, in the light of the above, do we want to go in the future (A)?

- Where are we now (B)?
- How to best get from B to A?

It is disappointing that it has required this sense of continuing financial pressure to force organisations to go back to basics, but undoubtedly that can be a very healthy process. As organisations become larger and/or long established there is always a danger that their very existence becomes an end in itself. Their initial 'raison d'être' becomes lost in the mist of time. This process is exacerbated where the financial discipline inherent in having to deliver a profit to make a living and/or satisfy shareholders is not uppermost. Where the budgetary process is felt to be vital and the questions listed earlier are being seriously addressed, it forces the organisation to be very clear about what its long-term objectives and short-term priorities need to be. A key point here is that those long-term objectives may well change over a period of time, particularly when one addresses the question 'where do we best add value?'. In a rapidly changing world it is not just what we can do that is changing. At least as crucial is the change in people's expectations. This is particularly so in large areas of the service sector, and health is a prime example of this.

The role of strategic management ultimately is to determine the direction of travel for an organisation, taking account of the key internal and external factors impacting upon it, i.e. to determine the 'direction we are going'. The budgetary process can assist very much in this thinking. All too often in the past either this thinking has not taken place or, perhaps more worrying, it has tended to be unfocused and general rather than specific. Budget debates force hard choices. These debates can, if used properly, help to tease out underlying issues and/or differences in perceptions within organisations.

The only way to achieve clarity around an organisation's strategy is to focus those earlier questions in the real world of difficult choices. These choices recognise explicitly a number of concepts, including:

- *Opportunity costs* Doing a particular thing prevents you doing something else – you have lost the opportunity to do X by doing Y.
- *Effectiveness* Using the minimum output to achieve the maximum benefit as determined by our objectives, in other words 'actively doing the things we need to achieve our objectives for the minimum input'.
- *Efficiency* Doing whatever we do at the best possible ratio of outcome to effort. However, efficiency is only worthwhile

if the outcome is broadly in line with the objectives, i.e. it is *effective*. Efficiency of itself cannot be an end. It is only a means of achieving an end.

Once the debate on setting a budget has determined the organisation's key objectives and clarified how it intends to deliver these objectives in as effective and efficient a way as possible, the budgetary control process should help to ensure that the organisation's focus is maintained. The reality is that to some extent this is an iterative process. The availability of resources, and the efficiency with which they can be used will clearly change over time. The budgetary control process will, therefore, act at two levels: (a) as a means of monitoring the continuing efficiency with which objectives are achieved; and (b) over the longer term as a means of checking out the original assumptions made about the direction of travel. This can be at the strategic level of bringing into question the very assumptions that were made about, for example, where the organisation best adds value, or at the tactical level of deciding how best to progress towards agreed objectives. All good strategic planning entails a continuing reiteration of the questioning approach epitomised earlier. The budgeting process can help.

A note of caution does, however, need to be struck. The process itself will not automatically lead to this continuing evaluation of strategic intentions. The organisation's culture needs to be open, flexible, strategic and evaluative. The budgeting discipline can then facilitate the process. Without these features the process could actually encourage the focus on the short term. There may still be an emphasis on efficiency, but it could be wrongly focused and eventually counter-productive to the achievement of the organisation's overall objectives.

As with most of the tools, and financial management is no exception, it is the hands holding the instruments that are the most important elements in achieving a good outcome.

In summary then we have described:

- how money is fed through the health system to fund the delivery of service at a local level on behalf of national government;
- efforts that have been made to achieve a greater level of equity of access to these funds;
- the considerable issues that still need to be visited to ensure equity at individual practice level;
- the clearer links contracting has established between funding and the delivery of service;

- description of terms including: capital, revenue, capital charges, EFL, PFI, 'cost per case', 'block', 'fixed and variable', 'marginal', ECRs, break-even and ratio/return; and finally
- how the budgeting process can help an organisation to clarify its thinking about its key objectives.

Managing a budget effectively is done in partnership with all groups of staff who contribute to the patient experience. Working together will ensure that resources as used to their optimum to ensure the best available care.

References

Department of Health and Social Security (1980) Inequalities in health: report of a Research Working Group (The Black Report). London: HMSO.

Department of Health (1997) The new NHS: modern, dependable. London: The Stationery Office.

Department of Health (1998) Our healthier nation – a contract for health. London: The Stationery Office.

Department of Health (1999) Saving lives: our healthier nation. London: The Stationery Office.

The business of finance

Application 6:1   *Julie Gray*

Financial issues in the health service

In Chapter 6, Con Egan has given a brief overview of financial issues in the health service, and outlines why it is so important that clinical professionals as well as professional accountants understand the principles behind, and the practice of, resource management. In this application, Julie Gray, who is sister in charge of the Pre-operative Assessment Clinic in Bradford, puts some of these principles into practice as she prepares an option appraisal considering different ways of using resources in order to make better use of facilities, and thus provide a better service for patients. This application is a summary of the full option appraisal, which was originally prepared whilst undertaking study for the Diploma in Health Services Management. The recommendation of Option B was accepted.

The Pre-operative Assessment Clinic (PAC) was set up in the Bradford Hospitals NHS Trust in existing accommodation, within a tight budget. An average of 600 patients, who have been listed for elective surgery, now attend the PAC for assessment each month.

The clinic has developed as part of the Trust's business plan in response to demand for services, and is a valuable asset to the Trust. It facilitates best use of general surgical, urology and orthopaedic beds and optimises theatre time. Although the clinic runs efficiently and effectively and represents value for money for the Trust, two additional services have been introduced; this has put pressure on the space. For the clinic to be even more efficient, a review of the available resources has been undertaken with a view to using the accommodation to its maximum potential. It has been estimated that for approximately £4300, an unused bathroom could be converted, and necessary equipment bought.

For the Trust, the activities of the PAC represent good practice and value for money. By assessing patients' suitability for elective surgery beds can be used efficiently, theatre lists can be filled to their optimum and patients replaced onto lists to cover cancellations, thus providing a quality service for users. If theatre lists run to maximum capacity this assists in keeping waiting list figures down and is more attractive to the Primary Care Groups who commission services from the Trust.

Clinical governance, described in the English White Paper 'The New NHS: Modern, Dependable' (Department of Health 1997) requires all staff to be accountable, and to improve quality of service provision by maximising resources. The aims of the PAC are to:

- identify patients who are unfit for elective surgery,
- assist in waiting list management,
- identify nursing problems prior to admission/implement plan of care,
- utilise beds efficiently,
- cut down on number of patients cancelled on day of admission, and
- act as an information source for patients and carers.

The staffing levels are shown in Table 6.1.1.

Two additional activities instigated within the PAC in 1999 have had an effect on clinic space utilisation: these are a waiting list initiative and a post-discharge follow-up clinic.

Table 6.1.1 Pre-operative Assessment Clinic staffing levels

Grade	WTE
H	1.00
G	2.00
D	4.93
C	0.86
A	2.23
Clerical	1.00
Clerical trainee	1.00
Total	**13.02 WTE**

The waiting list initiative was set up in January 1999 in order to reduce the general surgical waiting lists to meet contracts and waiting time standards. Until the end of March, extra theatre lists were carried out at weekends and during the week, where possible, and involved approximately 700 patients, all of whom passed through the PAC in addition to the normal monthly patient allocation.

The initiative was led by myself, the PAC sister and service nurse managers responsible for surgery and theatres. As the initiative progressed, the processes were reviewed in the light of the experience, and resulted in the current space being used in a different way.

Later in the same year, a nurse-led post-discharge follow-up clinic was instigated, which, whilst being a very successful and appropriate service, further encroached upon the space in the PAC.

MAXIMISING RESOURCES IN THE PAC

It is important to have clear outcomes in mind when seeking to use resources to their maximum. In consultation with relevant colleagues, the eight criteria were identified (Box 6.1.1).

The next step was to consider the options available to us to best achieve those eight criteria. In line with best practice, we aimed to have at least three options to consider, including a 'do nothing' option as a benchmark, in order that we might present a costed appraisal to management, and show a robust audit trail. We utilised a simple management tool – the Tartan Grid – to present an

---

Box 6.1.1 Eight criteria to be used when maximising the resources in the PAC

1. Improved working environment
2. Re-utilisation of resources
3. Waiting list management
4. Service development
5. Patient comfort/safety
6. Patient's Charter standards
7. Security of medical notes/computer
8. Improved utilisation of space

Delivering the business

objective, numerical representation of best use of precious resources.

Three options emerged:

- Option A – 'Do nothing'
- Option B – Refurbish bathroom, purchase new equipment
- Option C – Replace equipment only.

Option A – 'do nothing'

This option examines the implications of making no change to the utilisation of resources in the PAC. There are no advantages to this option. The service will develop, but space will remain limited and thus patients will wait a little longer than necessary.

Normally, there are five members of staff on duty at any one time who are able to assess patients, but currently there are only four assessment areas. This results in waste of a very valuable and expensive resource, and thus in lost opportunity costs.

Option B – refurbish bathroom, purchase new equipment

In this option, old sanitary ware would be removed from an unused bathroom and adjoining shower room to create extra office space for waiting list management. New equipment would be purchased to equip the extra assessment space.

This will result in a better environment and use of space, and thus better utilisation of resources, including nursing staff. Patient waiting times would be reduced, as five nurses will be assessing patients, rather than four. The equipment discarded from the PAC can be used effectively in other areas.

The above option will address:

- service development and waiting list management
- Patient's Charter standard (outpatient clinic waiting times).
- clinical governance framework
- service agreements with Primary Care Groups and the Health Authority.

Financial issues in the health service

195

Option C – replace equipment only

This option involves replacing equipment to allow an extra assessment area, but the unused bathroom would not be refurbished. Thus a potential office facility would be lost, and space would not be fully utilised.

COST IMPLICATIONS

It is important to present ideas with cost implications, and those of the three options are detailed in Table 6.1.2. When identifying costs, hidden costs and opportunity costs must be considered, as well as the actual costs of equipment etc. Option B emerged as the preferred option as all criteria are met.

Some equipment in the PAC can be used by the post discharge clinic; this will save money. The bath will be re-installed in another area.

IN CONCLUSION

The work carried out in the PAC is ongoing, thus the capital investment has significant cost benefits, and has the

---

Table 6.1.2   Cost implications of the three options

Option A
This involves no initial capital layout but lack of investment will result in lost opportunity costs and lack of scope for development. Also, the bathroom may require maintenance, resulting in a cost which will not attract direct benefit.

Option B
Cost of stripping out fixtures and fittings,
making good the surfaces, re-decoration and re-carpeting:

		£3500 + VAT
Equipment purchase – chair		£498 + VAT
trolley		£296 + VAT
	Total	**£4294 + VAT**

Option C
The purchase of a chair and trolley only as above:

Total	**£794 + VAT**

potential to make a real contribution to the quality of the patient experience, and the business of the Trust by:

- enabling the unit to continue to develop cost effectively as per Trust business plan,
- offering value for money,
- providing an area which offers adequate space for the projected throughput of patients, thus ensuring a safer environment, and
- providing an area conducive to the comfort and wellbeing of patients and staff.

Chapter **Seven**

Controlling the budget – setting the budget within resource

Rose Stephens, Julia Bradbury, Richard Romaniak

OVERVIEW

The budgetary control process is crucial to ensure effective management of revenue and capital budgets. In this chapter Rose Stephens, Julia Bradbury and Richard Romaniak discuss the routine processes managers carry out when planning the management of resources for the service for which they are responsible. They describe clearly, with examples, some dilemmas and choices managers face daily, and give

Delivering the business

background information about the processes involved. You will see from this chapter and from Con Egan's chapter (Chapter 6) the links between an individual organisation and the wider context of the NHS as a whole, and how each organisation must plan to meet its own population. Whilst, as Stephens, Bradbury, Romaniak and Egan note, the NHS is moving away from the annual contracting process, it is still important to consider a 12-month cycle of financial management so that firm controls can be applied on daily spending. The financial planning processes sit within the overall business planning processes described by Linda Terry in Chapter 4.

The NHS receives funding in the same way as other government departments: through the annual Treasury funding review (see Chapter 6). This annual cycle of funding meant that long-term strategic planning was underdeveloped, but for the short and medium term decision-making process, it was easier to adopt a clearly understood and relatively consistent approach. The new Labour administration, which was elected into power in May 1997, has acknowledged this weakness, and has identified a more strategic role for commissioners, and introduced Health Improvement Programmes (see Chapter 2).

THE BUSINESS PLANNING CYCLE

In order to plan service delivery and development around short-term resource allocation, health service organisations have developed a framework usually referred to as the 'business planning cycle' (see Chapter 4). The outcome of the business planning cycle determines the overall funding available to the organisation and forms the basis upon which individual service budgets are set.

The business planning process begins early in the financial year when national and regional guidelines are published which set the framework for commissioning organisations to work within. The guidelines act as a framework within which commissioners develop their purchasing plans for the following year. The commissioners signal their plans to providers through the issuing of formal purchasing intentions.

'The new NHS', with its emphasis on partnerships, has moved away from the formal annual contracting arrangements of the internal market of the 1990s by establishing 3-year service agreements, which encourage the development of partnerships. Providers will have developed their own corporate and departmental business plans in line with their strategic direction and these will need to be reviewed in the light of the commissioners' purchasing intentions. For example the commissioner may view that waiting lists are too long in ophthalmology and may indicate their intention to switch their contracts to another provider if improvements are not made. This has implications for the organisation, and the causes need to be analysed. If it is a resource issue, then a source of funding will need to be identified. This could be either from the commissioner or from a reallocation of internal resources.

Once priorities have been agreed with the commissioners then the provider needs to identify the resources required to deliver the specified levels of service. This will mean that some services will require an increased level of resource whilst others will need to release savings. It is usually the case that as part of the contracting process the commissioner is required to demonstrate efficiency savings. The commissioner will pass on part of this target through its contracts to the provider units. These efficiency savings will need to be taken into account when allocating resources to individual departments and services.

Thus the link is made between the level of resource available for departmental budgets and the planning process. Additional resource can be obtained normally only either through negotiation with the commissioner or internally generated by the provider through efficiencies.

Having determined the level of resource available to set individual budgets, the next step is to determine which method of budget setting it is most appropriate to adopt. There are three main approaches, each having advantages and disadvantages, which are examined now.

BUDGETING TECHNIQUES

There are three recognised techniques used in the NHS today (Box 7.1). Each of the three techniques is explored, and their respective strengths and weaknesses debated.

Box 7.1 Three approaches to budgeting in the NHS

1. Incremental budgeting
2. Zero-based budgeting
3. Activity-based budgeting

Incremental budgeting

This process uses historical information as a basis to prepare future budgets. Its starting point is the use of the previous year's budget, which forms the baseline for the following period. Any non-recurring elements are then deducted from this baseline. A non-recurring cost is an item purchased in one financial year only as a 'one off', for example funding of sessions requiring extra theatre staff associated with a waiting list initiative will be non-recurring.

The process takes account of any recurrent variances that occurred during the previous period and, having extrapolated them, reflects them in the following period. A recurring variance is expenditure incurred which is not currently budgeted for but which is expected to continue in the future. An example of this would be where the budget has been set for a consultant at the first incremental point of the scale, and he or she has received the annual increment, causing a budgetary variance. The consultant will continue to be paid this extra sum so it is an unavoidable cost and needs to be included in the budget.

Incremental budgeting also adapts the budget to take into account management plans. For example the extension of a day ward into an overnight facility which will require an additional budget setting for staff and enhancements associated with night duty, as well as budget planning to account for extra equipment etc. needed as a result of 24-hour service.

Inflation is accounted for using the incremental approach, therefore budgets are increased for pay awards and for any increase in non-pay inflation. Efficiency gains which recognise that over time more output can be achieved through the same level of resource, can be built into budgets.

Incremental budgeting is the method most commonly used in the NHS. As with the other budget setting techniques, it has advantages and disadvantages (Box 7.2).

Setting the budget within resource

> **Box 7.2** Incremental budgeting: advantages and disadvantages
>
> Advantages
> 1. It is a simple method to understand
> 2. Calculation is straightforward
> 3. It uses the minimum of management time
> 4. Its starting point is a base which has proved to be realistic for a given level of activity
>
> Disadvantages
> 1. The use of a historical base may allow inefficiencies and deficiencies to be hidden, as the process does not require the use of past resources to be justified.
> 2. There is no direct link between the level of funding and contracted activity levels. Budgets are often rolled forward from year to year without direct connection to the levels of activity that the budget is supporting.

Zero-based budgeting

This techniques requires that the budget for any given level of activity be calculated from scratch. Historic levels of funding and financial performance are only used for providing a perspective or reference point. All input costs are completely re-evaluated to construct a fresh budget for each activity undertaken by the organisation. For example, this may mean that based on occupancy levels a decision is taken to reduce the bed base in a particular specialty and therefore reduce the staffing levels, even though activity levels are the same as for the previous period.

The methodology for zero-based budgeting requires four key stages to be followed. The first stage involves identifying the quantity and quality of each service or activity provided by a department. For example, this may mean that 500 hip replacements are to be undertaken using a specified type of implant and that the maximum waiting time for an operation will be 6 months. The second stage identifies what resources are required to ensure that each service produces the required results. Using the previous example it will be necessary to consider all of the following:

- Number and staffing of outpatient clinics
- Number of theatre lists required based on length of time in theatre

- Composition of the theatre team
- Grade of medical staff
- Required number of beds based on length of stay
- Ward nursing establishment
- Ward and theatre consumable items
- Support from other departments, e.g. radiology and physiotherapy
- Hotel services, e.g. catering
- Administrative input.

The next stage is to ensure that the budget holder understands the budget and accepts ownership. This is achieved through ensuring appropriate involvement at all stages of the budget-setting process. Finally, it will be necessary to implement appropriate management changes to facilitate the revised budgetary arrangements.

As with incremental and activity-based budgeting there are both advantages and disadvantages to the zero-based approach to budget setting (Box 7.3). The method is most useful for identifying the value of further additions to the budget associated with new developments.

Activity-based budgeting

This technique aims to ensure that resources match activity levels at budgeted and actual levels of output. Prior to the start of the financial period it is necessary to determine the unit of output for which a standard cost is to be developed. This could be the number of finished consultant episodes (FCFs) for

---

Box 7.3 Zero-based budgeting: advantages and disadvantages

Advantages
1. The process ensures that a realistic achievable budget is set
2. Inefficiencies can be more readily identified
3. The relationship between cost and activity is recognised
4. It is challenging and establishes financial and operational goals for performance improvement

Disadvantages
1. It is very time consuming to prepare with the appropriate level of accuracy and objectivity, especially if activity levels are uncertain or not static
2. It may be difficult to implement due to the changes required

---

> **Box 7.4** Activity-based budgeting: advantages and disadvantages
>
> Advantages
> 1. Activity and finance are linked in a specific and meaningful manner
> 2. The results are realistic in relation to activity levels
> 3. It is simple to adjust budgets to reflect changing activity levels
> 4. It is easier to interpret variations from budgets and assess whether they are cost or activity related
>
> Disadvantages
> 1. Changes to standard costs may not be recognised
> 2. Flexing of budgets may fail to take into account the funds available. This may lead to a false sense of security for the budget holder. It is therefore important that activity is controlled to ensure that only work which can attract additional income is performed
> 3. There is the implicit assumption that activity can be budgeted for at standard cost

example. The next stage is to decide on an expected activity level to use in order to determine the 'standard' cost. It is then necessary to establish what resources are required for each unit of activity, distinguishing between costs which are fixed and costs which are semi-variable, variable or stepped costs. Having established the resources required for a given level of activity the standard cost can now be calculated by dividing the total expected costs by the total expected activity.

The initial budget set at the start of the period is based on budgeted activity at the 'standard' cost for each unit of activity, for example consultant episodes or outpatient attendances. The standard cost and the level of activity can then be changed up or down (known as flexing the budget) during the year because of revised forecast activity. This enables the budget to reflect the current requirements of the departments. Box 7.4 summarises the advantages and disadvantages of this approach.

BUDGET SETTING AND COST IMPROVEMENT

The NHS continues to face a seemingly endless increase in demand for its services, partly brought about by demographics and partly by medical advances. The result of this is that the NHS now works in an environment where resources are limited and priorities have to be set.

Consequently the annual budget setting process is linked intrinsically to the annual cost reduction process as organisations have to review resource allocation to enable contracted activity to be delivered within contracted income. Cost reductions can be delivered either through reductions in expenditure or through income generation.

Cost reduction programmes need to be approached in a systematic way if they are to be successful and care should be taken in ascertaining which services are suitable for targeting in the short, medium and longer term.

Use of benchmarking information

One possible way of identifying suitable services is the use of benchmarking, which compares the costs of services with those of other organisations with similar profiles. This information helps to narrow the field and highlight services where there may be inefficiencies. It is important to recognise that whilst benchmarking is a useful tool, the statistics are based on information supplied by many different individuals who may have interpreted the questionnaires in different ways. It is therefore essential that the comparators are compatible, i.e. like is compared with like.

Use of internal performance indicators

Other useful performance indicators include bed occupancy and theatre utilisation statistics. A low level of occupancy, for example, may indicate that it would be possible to manage activity through a reduced bed base.

With cost reduction, as with budget setting, it is important that the budget holder is actively involved in the process in order to ensure ownership from the beginning and commitment to achievement of the targets.

MONITORING AND CONTROL

To maintain satisfactory budgetary performance there needs to be a clearly defined financial control mechanism. Budgets are

Setting the budget within resource

a form of performance measurement for managers. They can identify how well a department or service is performing in relation to the objectives it has been set and subsequently its contribution to the overall corporate plan. In such a context budgets and budgetary performance have a very important role to play.

Framework of partnership

A successful framework for budgetary monitoring and control does not treat budgets as an issue in isolation, as many factors can affect budgetary performance. Such issues can include activity, case-mix, quality, guidance from the government or other statutory bodies, commissioner decisions, recruitment issues; the list of factors is endless. It is the budget holders' duty to be aware of the influences on their area and ensure that the risks are minimised.

Budget monitoring needs to be a partnership between finance and the budget holder. Where there are issues outside the budget holder's immediate control which affect their budgets, such as new health and safety legislation, it is important that the organisation recognises them and thus can plan any changes in advance to minimise any impact there may be to both the service provided and to the financial position.

To ensure that the partnership is a successful one, clear objectives for the budget holder must be set. In financial terms the most important objective is to provide a balanced budget. The budget holder must therefore be aware of what resources they have at their disposal in terms of manpower, 'skill-mix' and numbers, in the non-pay budgets and what activity is expected to be delivered. Ideally, they will have been actively involved in setting these targets and will therefore be fully knowledgeable about what the budgets contain. Without this information there will be difficulties later on in the year, particularly if cost reductions are required and resources are stretched by pressures from increased activity.

To meet the financial targets a budget holder needs the information to demonstrate what the current position is and what is expected. Without this information on a regular basis the budget holders cannot monitor their performance and rectify problems that may arise. Therefore without adequate budget monitoring, budgetary control is weak and the risk of failing to meet performance targets is increased.

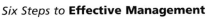

Budget monitoring

Senior managers in any organisation will monitor expenditure and performance. To ensure that the organisation meets its objectives, delegated management needs to be proactive in firstly monitoring performance and secondly undertaking remedial action when there is a risk that the planned position will not be achieved. Any budget requires regular, accurate information which can support its financial position. If information is not obtainable, there are weaknesses in the control processes in the area and there is an increased possibility of overspending.

The supportive information to assist effective budget monitoring needs to meet the following requirements:

- *Accurate* The information must be able to be validated. For instance, there are numerous checks in place in payroll office to ensure that staff are paid the correct sums. Most are recommended by internal audit, and are designed to ensure corporate governance and value for money
- *Timely* Information should ideally be available monthly and as soon as practicable. The earlier the information is available the better the decisions that can be made.
- *Relevant* Information needs to focus on the areas which affect the budget's performance. Extraneous information can be distracting and lead to indecision and poor choices.
- *Concise* Information needs to focus on only the key issues. It is difficult and time consuming to find the key points from a lengthy document when a summary would have identified the key points.
- *Understandable* This is very important and often undervalued. All managers of budgets need to be able to understand their financial statements. Without such knowledge, the ability to identify the causes of variances and the remedial actions to take is limited and therefore the financial risk is increased.

If the monitoring information does not fulfil these criteria, issues may not come to the budget holders' or the accountants' notice until it is too late for corrective action to be successful.

The budget holders have a responsibility to ensure that they have all the tools they require to monitor their budgetary performance effectively. They need to specify what information they need and what support they require to control their budget.

They need to understand their budgets and the assumptions made in their setting, otherwise they may be misled by variances occurring and make inappropriate decisions.

Budgetary controls

There needs to be a series of constraints in place to make it difficult and undesirable to overspend. Controls will vary from the physical controls preventing expenditure taking place to the reporting of budget performance to the board.

Physical controls

There are two main areas where a budget holder can incur expenditure, pay and non-pay. Pay is the area where traditionally the greatest number of constraints has been placed. There are two main reasons for this. First, pay accounts for approximately 70% of all NHS expenditure. Therefore, if there are strict controls on pay financial risk is minimised. Second, when expenditure is incurred on pay there will be a contract of employment involved. Employment law is such that redundancy costs can be significant, and this needs to be taken into account.

Physical controls on pay
The key to controlling pay is through the use of the staffing establishment. This should identify what number of staff are required and what skill-mix of staff is required to provide the level of service the commissioners require. It should be very specific and it should prevent pay exceeding the budgeted level. There are several advantages to utilising the staffing establishment in this way. It is widely used in the organisation and practical for all departments. There is plenty of validated and accurate information from the payroll system to support the budget position. It is also easy to understand and reasons for variances are identifiable. It can also clearly identify when there are problems with recruitment, which may result in the staffing levels being under establishment but with locum, bank or agency staff causing an overspend.

Physical controls on non-pay
For non-pay there can be a more flexible approach as it encompasses such a wide variety of items and areas. One of the most effective control measures is that of authorised signatories. A

Delivering the business

delegated budget holder may be authorised to sign invoices or order items worth up to say £500. For any items worth above this value a senior manager would need to authorise them. Another control can be set through the supplies system whereby a budget holder can only order items which are deemed appropriate for that department. So, for instance, a ward would not be expected to purchase laboratory equipment.

The most effective control overall on non-pay is through having a centralised supplies department. It is its role to ensure orders are placed correctly and that the organisation manages to get the best value for money possible. For larger items, such as a major piece of medical equipment, the most important controls are brought through effective business planning. Expensive items of equipment are purchased generally through capital funds which are separate from the revenue budgets of most budget holders. They can, however, have a major impact on the revenue budgets, through using different or more expensive consumables and by requiring new maintenance contracts. The business plan for the equipment must take into account the revenue consequences of the purchase, which must be found through either extra funding from commissioners or from internal efficiencies.

Remedial actions

With all budgets there are risks that at some stage they may overspend. When such an event occurs it is the budget holder's duty to address the situation, with the assistance of their accountant. The first action always is to investigate the cause of the variance and to ascertain if the problem is likely to continue or not. Once this has been established an action plan is required. Generally if there is an overspend there are two main causes: either the plan is faulty or there are problems with expenditure.

Options to address the plan

If the variation has been caused by the plan being at fault, action needs to be taken to get the plan in line with the expected situation. For instance if the operating theatres had their budget set on the assumption that there would be 1000 hip replacements in a year when the commissioners are expecting 1500, the budget, and therefore the plan, would have a shortfall of 500 hip

209

replacements. In these circumstances, the plan and/or the budget may be revised.

This is not always a straightforward process and emphasises the importance of full participation in the budget setting process as inadequacies in the annual budget are often difficult to resolve in a year. This is particularly true when there are internal efficiencies to be met, reducing any scope for flexibility. If no more resource can be put into the budget a review of the entire service may be required to balance the budget. This may mean addressing the expenditure of the department through altering the working practices, changing ordering patterns or any other measure which can release internal efficiencies.

Options to address expenditure issues

If overspend is caused by problems with expenditure the one option that is not available is to do nothing! One of the key management goals is to break even. The actions available vary depending on the causes of the variance and the type of budget. An overspend could be due to a change in unit cost, for example, photocopying charges increasing from 3p to 4p a copy. Alternatively the overspend could be caused by a change in activity, for example the number of copies taken has risen from the expected 10 000 per month to 12 000. Various options are available to resolve the situation.

- Cut the spending in the problem area back to budget. This would mean that if more than expected was being spent on photocopying, expenditure must be reduced until parity is restored. This could be achieved by rationing the usage of the facility (manage activity down to target), or by renegotiating a cheaper contract (reduce unit cost down to plan). This approach can work on less complex budgets. However, it may not be possible or desirable to cut back on the expenditure upon an individual item, so other methods must be considered.
- Cut the spending down in the department to budget level but not necessarily in the problem area. A department's budgets generally incorporate more than one budget line and so a more flexible approach may be taken. In the example of photocopying costs it may be possible to purchase the paper and stationery cheaper by using an alternative supplier, or by purchasing in bulk in conjunction with other departments or even organisations in order to get the best prices.

- Transfer budget from another area. A budget holder may be in charge of several departments and may have some funding available in one area to put into an underfunded budget. This is known as virement. The risk here is that short-term funds can be found to hide long-term problems. Reasons for variances need to be tackled quickly to ensure that long-term overspends do not occur.
- Find a long-term solution. It may be that in the short term a balanced budget cannot be achieved. It is vital that a long-term plan is drawn up quickly to address the situation. If it is not, there is the potential for resources being moved from the ideal (direct patient care) to the lower priority areas such as overheads.

Factors to take into account when addressing overspends

When identifying the actions required to resolve an overspent budget it is important to take into account practical constraints. The issues to take into account include the following:

- How controllable are the costs? Not all items are within the budget holders' full control for example. The costs in operating theatres can be influenced greatly by changes in case-mix that cannot be fully controlled or planned by the budget holder. It is important that these areas are identified and the risks are minimised through having excellent reporting systems to identify issues the moment they arise. It is equally important that all controllable items have rigid systems in place, so that avoidable problems do not occur.
- What is the sensitivity of the item? Is the item easily affected by factors out of your control? Is it affected by several factors? Is it an item that is indispensable or only available from one supplier thus the price is not affected by competition?
- How much time is left to find a solution? If an overspend occurs late in the financial year it is much more difficult to balance the position than if it happens earlier. This places great importance on reliable and timely monitoring to ensure that any problems are identified quickly and are not left unnoticed until it is too late to rectify them.
- The consequence for future years must be considered: careful and thorough examination of the circumstances will minimise the future impact of the current problem.

211

Setting the budget within resource

- Is there a possibility of virement or of carry forward of monies? In the health service the accounts are closed at the end of the financial year and underspends are lost, and thus this makes carrying forward of money difficult. However, if the organisation overspends in one financial year they have to plan to produce a balanced position either in the proceeding year or within 3 years, depending upon the size of the problem. This may leave some scope for longer term solutions to be found when all efforts made in the current year to balance have been unsuccessful. A budget holder can transfer funds between some budgets but must be wary of hiding any long-term problems by 'quick-fix' solutions.

ANNUAL BUDGETING CYCLE – SOME PROBLEMS

There are a number of problems associated with setting budgets on an annual basis.

Use it or lose it

Annual budgets reinforce the fact that much planning in the NHS is done on a short-term basis. Along with other government departments the NHS operates on a cash basis and therefore does not have the flexibility to carry forward savings from one year to the next although this is being addressed at strategic level. This method of funding creates a perceived disincentive at departmental level to spend only what is needed as savings are effectively lost to the budget holder.

Inflexibility

It is expected that organisations will balance their books every year although recently there has been some relaxation in this rule. This means that when an organisation is faced with an unexpected financial problem they have to find a solution very rapidly and this can lead to inappropriate decisions being made.

Timing of budget setting

Budgets have to be agreed quite early on in the financial year, often before the outcomes of contract negotiations are known.

This means that they become reliant on assumptions that may not be consistent with the organisation's objectives for the period. Where income is set to be lower than budget expenditure this leads to the need for rapid cost reduction plans and cuts in budgets being made in an unplanned way. As the longer term agreements are established, this should minimise this difficulty. For example, savings could be made by reducing a budget that underspent in the previous financial year on the basis that it is a quick way of balancing the books even though comparisons show this to be a well-managed and efficient area. Services that are inefficient may thus be overlooked.

Resource constraints

Whatever approach is taken when setting budgets, either incremental, zero-based or activity-based, it is a time-consuming process. The need to set budgets annually means that it is usually the incremental approach that is adopted. This often means that there is a failure to take account of changes that have affected the organisation, such as reduced length of stay in a particular specialty and their impact on the need for resources. This can partially be overcome by ensuring that there is a clear link between the business planning process and the budget setting process. However, whilst funding is agreed on an annual basis, time constraints will always be a problem.

Boom and bust

There is often an expectation that organisations can increase and decrease their capacity at short notice. In an organisation such as the NHS which has a large number of fixed and semi-fixed costs this can be problematic. However the annual budget setting process will still be required to deliver a balanced plan.

Clearly budget setting in this environment is not easy but the limitations of the annual budget process can be mitigated by ensuring that 'best practice' is used for the budget setting process. As the NHS moves towards 3-year agreement cycle, rather than 1-year contracts, it is likely still that organisations will consider their operational budgets within an annual framework, whilst working strategically to the 3-year perspective.

Good communication between the finance department and budget holders is essential. This will ensure that all factors which might lead to variances from plan are identified at an

Setting the budget within resource

early stage and plans can be formulated to generate savings to cope with any anticipated overspends. The key issue is to ensure that both the finance staff and the budget holders have a good understanding of all the issues, including the service delivery problems and the financial framework that must be operated within. If this understanding is achieved, mutual trust and commitment to the achievement of the organisation's objectives will become the norm.

Controlling the budget

**In this case study Rose Stephens and Julia Bradbury
outline a routine management challenge, and describe
how teamwork and appropriate planning processes can
be used to meet the needs of the service.**

This case study has been based in an acute hospital setting,
although the issues identified could easily be encountered
in community environments and indeed, to a degree, in the
private sector. It identifies a situation where hospital and
nursing management need to take action in a proactive
manner to avoid a serious financial problem. It is these
issues that senior nurses and managers have to face on a
regular basis in the NHS of today.

The NHS, like most organisations is open to market
forces. The key pressures in the NHS are increasing demand
and increased expectations. These arise from a number of
sources: from the public through greater awareness and
generally improved standards of living, from the
government through targeted funding initiatives and
patient charter standards, and from clinicians and general
practitioners through greater involvement in the
development and management of health care provision.
These pressures inevitably are leading to conflicts on a daily
basis for most health care professionals.

THE ISSUES

As the reshaping of the health service takes a high priority
for the current government it was one of their first tasks to

lay down their view of how the NHS should be structured. An early change was focused upon the GP fundholding scheme being disbanded and replaced in England by the Primary Care Group format. The new system will require providers of health care to become more responsive to the needs of the local population as commissioning becomes more than ever primary care driven. Similar arrangements exist in Scotland, Wales and Northern Ireland, and these are addressed in Chapter 2.

The government has made waiting list sizes and waiting times one of its key priorities. In the first full year this manifested itself into two specific targets for acute providers: first, to ensure that no patient should wait more than 12 months for elective surgery (excludes certain specialist services) and secondly, that in total, the number of patients on waiting lists should not rise above the numbers on lists as at 1 May 1997.

The targets set by the government to reduce waiting lists and waiting times present the management of provider organisations with some major challenges, as at the same time as being asked to increase activity, they must still demonstrate efficiency savings. Also, as yet there has been no relaxation in the rule to break even each year. A further problem is that year on year emergency activity has been increasing and resource allocation has not kept pace.

This case study looks at how an acute provider may respond to this particular conflict.

HITTING THE WAITING LIST TARGETS AND BREAKING EVEN

The local district general hospital has worked together with the local Health Authority to agree its targets for the coming financial year. This plan incorporates both finance and activity and, as a result of the government emphasis on waiting times and waiting list sizes, the hospital has been asked to perform an additional 1000 operations across various specialties. The government has indicated that it does not expect to pay more than £500 per case for this activity. The hospital has identified that the normal average price it would charge for these operations would be £750 per case.

> **Box 7.1.1**   The planning process: points to consider
>
> - Total cost of delivery: the 1000 cases must not exceed 1000 × £500, i.e. £500 000
> - Ability to cope with emergency activity must not be affected and indeed plans need to be sufficiently flexible to allow for a rise during the year
> - The performance standards agreed to in existing contracts must still be met, e.g. treatment to take place within 3 months of listing
> - Core income flows need to be maintained. Careful planning of case mix will be needed to ensure that existing contracts can still be met in full
> - As all assets (staff and facilities) are generally used to maximum capacity a clear strategy to increase capacity needs to be identified

Clearly, the hospital will have to draw up a careful operational and financial plan before agreeing to undertake this work to ensure that it can reconcile its two conflicting targets of breaking even and delivery of the agreed level of service. The hospital must ensure that the points listed in Box 7.1.1 are considered in the planning process.

The planning process needs to be multidisciplinary with input essential from clinicians, operational managers, finance, contracting and information services to ensure that all the above points are covered. It is of particular importance to involve clinical staff in the early stages as it is likely that they will be required to undertake flexible working patterns if the plan is to succeed.

THE DETAILED PLAN

It has been identified that 300 of the 1000 cases can be designated as general surgery. The budget holder for this area formed a working group to look at the operational and resource issues which arise. Unfortunately the timescales allowed by the purchaser do not allow the hospital to establish a detailed case-mix for this work and consequently the resources required will be identified assuming the average. The budget holder has identified that the team should consist of herself, the senior nurse for the area, the theatre manager, the senior general surgeon, the senior anaesthetist and her finance manager. The plan that they develop will be shared with all other departments to ensure that they can identify the resources they may require to support the front line services in delivering the additional work. It will be important to ensure that budget holders look only at what resource is required to deliver the plan and do not seek to rectify any current underlying or perceived problems.

The working group identified the following areas to look at:

- How many theatre lists will be required?
- Will the bed base be adequate?
- Will any additional equipment be required?
- Consult with support services to identify their issues.

The results of this groundwork have revealed the following:

- An additional theatre list will be required every week for the next 50 weeks based on six cases per list, which hospital data shows to be the average number of cases per list. The senior surgeon and theatre manager believe that this is a reasonable assumption. Due to staffing constraints this list will have to take place on Saturday mornings.
- Based on average length of stay the bed-base will not be adequate and it has been decided to overcome this by re-opening an extra three beds.
- The additional theatre list will have to take place in a decommissioned theatre and therefore the theatre manager has provided a list of essential equipment.
- Support services have indicated that they will need extra resource to support this activity, primarily because it is taking place out of core hours.

IDENTIFICATION OF RESOURCE REQUIREMENTS

The next stage in the process is for the budget holder to identify what resources, if any, will be needed to support the increased capacity. In deciding what resources are needed and whether the plan is operationally feasible the budget holder must take account of whether the funding is going to be available on a recurrent basis. For example, the theatre manager must assess whether the extra list can be covered within the existing staff hours available to her or whether it will require overtime to be worked or new staff employed. The ward sister will need to work with the budget holder to assess the impact on staffing of opening the three extra beds.

The cost of the equipment will need to be identified and so will any associated capital charges (items over £5000) and maintenance costs. If a major piece of capital equipment is required there could be a significant lead-in time before this becomes available.

Support services will need to undertake a similar exercise.

Once all the costs and operational issues have been identified, a decision can be taken whether or not to proceed. If the costs identified are in excess of the funding available a thorough review will need to be undertaken in conjunction with the other specialties to establish what if any savings can be made. For example, there may be duplications in the resources identified, i.e. both orthopaedics and general surgery may have identified the need for an additional consultant anaesthetist who would not be used to capacity in either area and could, in fact, cover both specialties.

REVIEW AND IMPLEMENTATION OF THE PLAN

If a decision were taken to proceed, the funding available would need to be allocated to budget holders based on the requirements identified by them in the plan. It would then be necessary to monitor carefully the expenditure incurred in relation to the activity achieved. In order to assist the monitoring process it is important to ensure that funding allocated is clearly identifiable and does not disappear into the overall budget; ideally funding should only be made available once the expenditure has been committed. Any variation from the plan both in terms of expenditure or activity needs to be investigated on a timely basis and action identified to rectify the situation. Ideally a

Controlling the budget

contingency should be included to acknowledge that some things are unpredictable.

In order to ensure that efficiency is maximised, at the end of the period covered by the plan a review should be undertaken. This review will cover both the operational and financial performance against plan. The process will ensure that lessons are learnt and pitfalls avoided in the future.

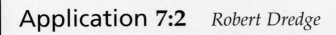

Application 7:2 *Robert Dredge*

Reading the budget

In this application, Robert Dredge shows the links between the individual ward budget and the overall financial well being of the Trust. This information is achieved as a result of the activities you have read about earlier in this chapter.

A budget describes the amount of resources allocated to achieve a predetermined set of outputs and describes both income or expenditure. Budgets are expressed in terms of money and number of people available as a resource. Normally a budget is set for one complete financial year, but can be adjusted during the year if circumstances change.

Budgets are compared against actual performance and the variances analysed to determine if any action is needed to stay within the limits of the budget. The most usual period of comparison is the calendar month, although some organisations use 4-week periods, and some, where trends and control is critical, may report weekly.

STRUCTURES OF BUDGETS

Budgets are organised to reflect the management, control and authority hierarchy of an organisation. For a hospital operating a system of devolved management (and by definition devolved budgetary control) the model will be something like:

Trust Board
|
Clinical directors
|
Directorate subdivisions
|
Operational units

The following case study demonstrates examples of how this structure is interpreted into a budget and shows its lines of accountability.

BOARD LEVEL

The Board will need to know the overall position of its various accountable units, and the information is likely to be prepared in a format such as that shown at Table 7.2.1. A minus sign before a figure indicates an underspend in this example. This statement shows an overspend, in total, of £266 000 to date.

The Board will have agreed the budgets for each of its directorates and divisions (management, estates, etc.). The annual budget will have been divided over each of the 12 accounting periods (months of the year). This division may have been in equal twelfths for items likely to occur evenly across the year, or may be more sophisticated to allow for:

● seasonal variations (e.g. energy costs are higher in winter than summer and so 40% of budget is put into months 1–6, 60% into months 7–12 based upon previous years usage);

Table 7.2.1 Month 11 board report (£'000)

Total directorate variance	Pay Annual budget £'000	Pay To-date variance £'000	Non-pay Annual budget £'000	Non-pay To-date variance £'000	Total variance £'000
Surgery	6732.1	−12.2	2001.0	−53.6	−65.8
Medicine	8672.6	−15.7	2628.7	284.9	269.2
Pathology	796.0	−20.3	1643.2	31.3	10.0
Total	6432.0	−210.0	26 400.0	476.0	266.0

Delivering the budget

- planned holidays (pay budgets could be adjusted if it is practical, for example, to shut theatres during August or over Christmas); and
- variations in the number of days per month (i.e. January is 31/365 of total, February 28/365, etc.) to give greater accuracy.

It does not really matter which method is used as long as the basis of the budget is known, and allowed for in assessing any trends in variance.

The overall position of the hospital is shown in the total variance figure in the bottom right hand column of Table 7.2.1. It is overspent by £266 000 at the end of Month 11 (February). The directorate analysis presented to the Board tells it where this overspend has come from, but it does not explain why it has arisen.

Let us focus on the medical directorate. The summary level report to the Board shows there to be:

- Pay underspend of £15 700
- Non-pay overspend of £284 900
- Total overspend of £269 200.

The reporting structure relating to this summary will consist of the various management and accountable units of the directorate. The budget reporting structure of the medical directorate could be something like that shown in Table 7.2.2. When presented, analysed and discussed at the

Table 7.2.2 The medical directorate: summary expenditure against budget

	Pay		Non-pay		Total	
	Annual budget £'000	Mth 11 variance £'000	Annual budget £'000	Mth 11 variance £'000	Annual budget £'000	Mnth 11 variance £'000
Acute nursing	3 106 976	32 118	209 704	34 269	3 316 680	66 387
Emergency nursing	926 644	22 936	34 771	−1409	961 415	21 527
Management	1 952 369	22 395	43 681	13 057	1 996 050	35 452
Departments	1 239 070	−63 809	822 025	25 765	2 061 095	−38 044
Care of the elderly	1 178 133	−6471	35 102	11 037	1 213 235	4566
Subtotal GU	269 413	−22 911	29 218	−12 063	298 631	−34 974
Subtotal blood	0	0	155 963	27 235	155 963	27 235
Bed hire	0	0	29 048	85 347	29 048	85 347
Drugs	0	0	1 269 213	101 640	1 269 213	101 640
Total	8 672 605	−15 742	2 628 725	284 878	11 301 330	269 136

directorate's business meeting this table begins to put some detail on the budget performance. The line by line analysis allows the Board to see that:

● The pay underspend is not consistent within the directorate. Three areas, departments, elderly and GU are underspending, whilst three others have overspends.
● Non-pay is overspending in all but two areas. The overspend ranges from £11 037 in care of the elderly to £101 640 in drugs.

This analysis gives some detail about the total position. It shows where, but not why, variances are occurring. In terms of managing a budget it indicates to the clinical director and his or her team the areas that need further investigation, and where possible corrective action needs to be taken. The major 'problems' (in financial terms) are the nursing and management overspends, and those of bed hire and drugs.

The next level of detail that should be provided is the individual ward/department analysis. Building on the example used above, the detail provided for acute nursing is shown in Table 7.2.3. The allocated budget and 'actual' position shows there to be both large over- and underspends on pay. The financial performance of the

Table 7.2.3 Acute nursing: ward by ward expenditure against budget

	Pay		Non-pay		Total	
	Annual budget £'000	Mth 11 variance £'000	Annual budget £'000	Mth 11 variance £'000	Annual budget £'000	Mnth 11 variance £'000
1	136 595	−28 184	12 674	5415	149 269	−22 769
2	359 516	17 198	28 171	4809	387 687	22 007
3	401 012	18 861	20 063	4604	421 075	23 465
4	400 222	−1728	24 851	3807	425 073	2079
5	399 026	18 177	27 875	2521	426 901	20 698
6	406 955	−14 933	29 749	−3225	436 704	−18 158
7	93 213	23 600	14 000	17 361	107 213	40 961
8	398 591	7250	25 439	−3099	424 030	4151
9	397 582	8303	23 836	835	421 418	9138
Nurse management	114 264	−16 426	3046	1241	117 310	−15 185
Subtotal acute nursing	3 106 976	32 118	209 704	34 269	3 316 680	66 387

wards is not consistent and this may suggest that some redeployment of budgets between wards could be helpful. Non-pay is almost consistently overspent.

There will be similar detailed reports for each of the areas within the directorate. Each of these reports tells the readers where the budget is allocated and where expenditure has arisen, but does not explain further about why these circumstances may have arisen.

THE NEXT LAYER OF INFORMATION

In order to understand 'the why' the reader needs information about staff numbers by grade, agreed establishment and the actual numbers of staff employed. This detail will show quickly if more or less staff have been employed than allowed for in the budget. It will give one easy explanation for an under- or overspend, but will not justify the variance. The reader also needs information about activity planned and achieved (number of cases, consultant episodes, etc.). If more patients have been treated than the budget assumed then overspends may be explained, but not necessarily justified.

CAPITAL EXPENDITURE

Capital is money allocated to carry out a specific 'one-off' project (see Chapter 6), and NHS central funding is determined by two sources:

- the regional office which agrees major schemes, funded on a 'scheme by scheme' basis, and
- the discretionary scheme, agreed locally from a block allocation, in agreement with the regional office.

The Trust may also choose to access the private finance initiative (PFI) (discussed in Chapter 6).

The capital programme and budget will need to be reported to the Board in such a way that it can be satisfied that:

- Schemes are not overspending
- Schemes are achieving their target timetables
- Future year capital is not overcommitted.

Reading the budget

Table 7.2.4 Capital budget (£'000)

Scheme	Spend projection			Spend to date	
	1998 £'000	1999 £'000	2000+ £'000	Plan £'000	Actual £'000
Major scheme					
Day unit	248	29	–	248	275
Maternity	128	50		128	56
Discretionary					
Ward upgrade	400	50	–	300	310
Outpatients upgrade	300	150	–	210	100
Car parking	250	–	–	250	236
Statutory standards	250	250	250	150	174
Medical equipment	300	500	500	450	410
Total	1876	1029	750	1736	1561

An example of a capital report format is shown in Table 7.2.4. This shows the Trust to have a capital budget, in total, of £1 876 000 for 1998. It also gives notice to the Board that it has agreed to have pre-committed £1 029 000 in 1999 and £750 000 in the year 2000. (These can, of course, subject to contractual commitments, be adjusted in these years.)

The planned spend in 1998, to date was £1 736 000, but only £1 561 000 has actually been spent. The main variances are in the maternity schemes and outpatients upgrade. The Board should seek an explanation for this.

A projected year-end position must be prepared to indicate whether any corrective action is needed now.

Chapter **Eight**

Cost-effective services

Eva Lambert

OVERVIEW

In this chapter Eva Lambert introduces and discusses the need for active management to ensure services provided by and for the NHS are cost-effective. Whilst most of these processes were introduced as a direct result of the introduction of the internal market, the concept and principle of accountable and effective resource management remains a key feature in health care today.

A simple definition of a cost-effective service is the provision of a service which meets the required standard at the least cost and representing best value. This is not the same as providing the cheapest – in fact there will be occasions when the least expensive option is not selected. When a competitive tendering exercise is undertaken and all the options have been evaluated, the decision may be made to recommend in-house services even though they are not the cheapest. The value attached to both continuity of services and good industrial relations can justifiably outweigh the benefit of cost savings where these are fairly small. Similarly, a value can and should be placed on the certainty of supply in particular critical areas and where this is justified this value will be included in the assessment of what is the best outcome in terms of overall value for money. The statutory duty of NHS organisations to ensure quality of service in addition to their duty to balance budgets and the announcement of the ending of compulsive competitive tendering in favour of 'Best Value' will pose some challenging dilemmas.

NON-CLINICAL SERVICES

The most common services to be subject to evaluation of cost-effectiveness have been those (historically) in domestic cleaning, catering and laundry. These were the first services to be subjected to compulsory competitive tendering.

Competitive tendering is the offering of an invitation to tender for the provision of a service or supply of goods, for which there is more than one possible provider, to a number of providers. These providers may then submit in detail a tender outlining how they will provide the service and at what cost. The tenders must all be submitted to the same specification, at the same time and in the same way. The tenders are then evaluated to establish the provider offering the best value for money. In order to ensure this exercise is undertaken, some goods and services must be subject to competitive tender – this is known as compulsory competitive tendering (CCT). There have been various other value-for-money initiatives which have added other services to the list but these have not been subject to compulsory competitive tendering. 'The NHS Plan' (Department of Health 2000) states that since the introduction of CCT and the internal market patients perceive a deterioration in cleanliness of hospitals. In September 2000 at the Labour Party Conference, the secretary of state announced the end of CCT in favour of the 'Best Value' approach used in local government.

CLINICAL SERVICES

There has been a number of initiatives which have sought to identify whether clinical services are cost-effective. Management budgeting in the early 1980s sought to provide individual clinicians with a budget for their clinical service and then to involve individual consultants as budget holders. The Resource Management Initiative (RMI) which began in 1986 moved away from simply providing cost information to providing clinical information to inform clinicians in their clinical decision making and to actively involve them in the management process. It was felt that if services were clinically effective they would be cost-effective. This initiative was, to a certain extent, overtaken by the reforms which introduced the internal market, which again sought to achieve cost-effectiveness using market principles. The White Paper 'The New NHS: Modern, Dependable' (Department of Health 1997) removes the operation of the internal market, and seeks to replace it with a managed market.

The involvement of clinicians in the management process has continued with the growth of clinical directorates as a model of management structure for NHS Trusts, and is strengthened further within the framework of clinical governance. The introductions of clinical audit and the clinical effectiveness initiatives, including the National Institute for Clinical Excellence (NICE), are current examples of efforts to ensure that services are effective. The measurement of whether clinical services are effective is extremely complex and many of the current initiatives will take many years to achieve results. There is a significant cost associated with the processes and the real value these processes have added has been questioned.

Nevertheless, clinical activities must continue to develop and change and current initiatives will seem mundane in a few years. It is important, therefore, that the effectiveness of clinical interventions continues to be assessed. The requirement within the English White Paper 'The New NHS: Modern, Dependable' (Department of Health 1997) for Trusts to embrace the concept of clinical governance, together with the establishment of a Commission for Health Improvement (CHI), indicates that the government continues to see this as a priority. There may be less emphasis, however, on testing services in a 'market' approach with the introduction of the Best Value initiative. It is only relatively recently that the suggestions of clinical services being subject to tender have been made and then only in clinical support services such as pathology. There has been considerable debate about whether or not clinical services should be subject to competitive tender. Some commentators feel the 'market' should determine the provider and the price, whilst others feel this is not appropriate for health care. In clinical services it is certainly more difficult for other providers to demonstrate they could provide the services at the standards required and with the certainty of supply. In most clinical areas there is considerable input from a range of professionals working together, in a variety of roles, as a multiprofessional team. In many clinical situations the service cannot be predicted because each individual patient has differing needs and the clinical autonomy must be considered. The Best Value initiative promises a more sensitive approach.

PURCHASE OF GOODS

The NHS is a multibillion pound organisation and although around 70% of its expenditure is on staff, around 30% is spent on goods, ranging from expensive high-tech equipment costing millions of pounds to the bulk purchase of bread at a few pence per loaf. The provision of both clinical and non-clinical services depends on a supply of goods at the right time, of the required standard and specification, and representing good value for money. Many goods are purchased through the NHS supplies service whose role is to ensure that the NHS has effective and cost-effective purchasing. Supplies staff provide some services to all NHS organisations and are linked together nationally to provide opportunities for bulk purchasing. A supplies catalogue is available showing goods and prices available.

Each NHS organisation has its own internal arrangements determining which staff have authority and responsibility to order goods. These rules will cover the purchase of both stock and non-stock goods. Stock goods are those goods which are purchased in sufficient quantities across the NHS to allow for them to be held either centrally, regionally or at the supplier's premises. Non-stock items are those not held in stock and which require one-off purchasing. Whenever goods are purchased there should be a competitive tendering exercise to ensure the best price is obtained. In the standing orders of all NHS organisations there will be rules determining the cost of a purchase, above which cost competitive tendering must be undertaken. There will also be limits below this when competitive quotations must be obtained. In all cases the aim is to ensure that the best price is obtained for the goods.

ENSURING COST-EFFECTIVE SERVICES

It is important to recognise that services provided are not automatically cost-effective. In the early years of competitive tendering many heads of services in domestic cleaning, catering and laundry felt somewhat affronted that the cost-effectiveness of their services should be questioned. This was understandable, but as many of these services had been developed over the years in an ad hoc way it is not surprising that in some cases the result was a range of fragmented services.

The starting point for any service evaluation is to specify the service required. This needs to be an agreed service specification. Normally, the head of the particular service defines the current service and then consults various users for their views. Alternatively, the user will define their service needs and then the professional head will ensure that this constitutes best practice. It is important that the outcome shows quite clearly:

● the existing service,
● any changes needed to comply with recommended standards, and
● any other change to meet users needs.

The existing budget will be based on the current service, and any changes that might affect resources used will need to be considered.

The process to arrive at the agreed specification will be an iterative one and will often be challenged by both user and provider in terms of what is needed and how it can best be provided. Often some degree of compromise is necessary to ensure legitimate needs can be met whilst not increasing the costs unnecessarily or impinging upon other priorities.

SERVICE REVIEW

Service reviews should take place against a detailed service specification that has been agreed with service users. An example is illustrated in Figure 8.1. Involving service users may highlight various tasks which could be linked together to improve the utilisation of staff time needed. For example, cleaning services provided at weekends and evenings often attract premium rates of pay and if these could be curtailed whilst still maintaining standards, this could lead to cost savings.

Cost-effective services

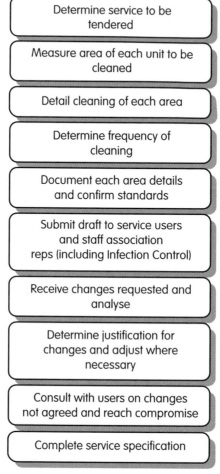

Figure 8.1 Service specification for domestic cleaning.

Challenge of any service provision is important. Simply accepting that the status quo is acceptable is not appropriate. There is always room for improvement in the provision of any service. Equally it is important that standards are not reduced to such a level that problems occur which may increase costs elsewhere. This could happen, for example, if cleaning frequencies were reduced to such an extent that there was an increase in cross-infection rates resulting in patients needing to stay in hospital longer.

It is always possible to spend more on a service but this must be evaluated to ensure that the extra cost adds sufficient extra value, and to ensure that other priorities are met. Failure to do this may result in the loss of opportunity costs. Using resources in one way is always at the expense of something else (i.e. money can only be spent once); this concept is known as opportunity costs. The opportunity to use resources in other ways should be considered as part of the overall evaluation of the service.

SERVICE INTEGRATION

Ward cleaning duties are now often combined with other duties, forming a 'housekeeper' role, and the member of staff is included as part of the ward team. Ward sisters usually welcome this as duties can then more easily be integrated into the general running of the ward. For the member of staff involved, this change of roles can provide increased job satisfaction. There have been examples of resistance from professional heads of domestic service as it can be seen as reducing their sphere of responsibility, but the gains have often proved to outweigh the losses.

It is important to ensure that the end users of the service are involved in the changes and are satisfied that the service provided in this way will meet their needs. It is also important to ensure that where these types of developments occur there is sufficient input from professional heads to ensure standards are met. Suitable monitoring arrangements should prevent any reduction in standards occurring.

BENCHMARKING

It is important to review internal specification standards vigorously. Ongoing review of all services as part of an overall continuous improvement programme will encourage everyone to accept change more readily. Reviewing a service against external data can introduce more challenge and encourage a more open approach when considering how the service could be provided.

Benchmarking is a process whereby organisations identify best performers and examine how such results are achieved, with a view to bringing their own performance into line with best practice identified. Benchmarking has become more popular over recent years. Simple cost comparisons can provide a starting point to indicate where there are major differences, but it is important then to check that the services being compared are similar. Benchmarking involves the identification of a number of

233

indicators which allow comparisons across similar services. Indicators will include such things as staff/workload ratios, staff/cost ratios, qualified/unqualified staff ratios, etc. Where similar services exist, heads of service can be encouraged to talk to colleagues to share good practice. There has been some reluctance to share information in the past due to the competitive atmosphere of the internal market, but with the move towards a spirit of partnership, this should be overcome.

MARKET TESTING

Market testing for some services has been in place for many years and is now undertaken on a regular basis. The process is part of standard business practice and allows comparisons of services provided in-house with those provided by private or other public sector providers. The process of various providers being required to provide details of how and at what price they can supply a particular service is more likely to lead to a radical review of provision. A detailed description of the process can be found later in the chapter.

CONTRACTING OUT

Contracting out a service means contracting with an external supplier for provision of a service. The process of market testing may or may not result in a service being 'contracted out'. In some cases the organisation may have taken a decision that provision of a particular service by the NHS is not part of their 'core business' and thus it will be contracted out. This will entail drawing up a detailed service specification, which will then be competitively tendered but without the submission of an in-house bid. The human resource implications are similar to those when the service is not won by in-house providers and are dealt with later in the chapter.

AUDIT COMMISSION

The Audit Commission is the statutory body whose main duties are to appoint auditors to local authorities and NHS Trusts, to ensure those bodies:

- comply with current legislation,
- prepare financial statements in line with legislation, and
- safeguard their organisations against fraud.

The Commission also undertakes value for money (VFM) studies across a sample of organisations and produces a report of its findings. These studies are designed to promote best practice in local government and NHS bodies to ensure economy, efficiency and effectiveness in the management and delivery of services. The auditors appointed by the Commission then undertake local audit studies to compare the organisation with the results of the national studies. These reports provide local management with information on their performance and what could be done to improve it to the level of the best performers.

AUDIT REPORTS

Audit reports are produced by the Audit Commission, the local external auditors and the internal auditors of the local NHS organisation. Each audit report must be acted upon by the relevant officers of the organisation. Audit reports will be submitted to the manager responsible for the appropriate area, together with recommendations for action, which are then converted into agreed objectives. Action on the results should be reported to the Audit Committee of the Trust or Health Authority whose responsibility it is to ensure the organisation responds appropriately to report recommendations.

ASSESSING VALUE FOR MONEY

Non-clinical goods and services

The provision of any service or the supply of any goods to the NHS must reflect value for money. It is particularly important because the funds utilised come from the public purse and the NHS must always be accountable for their use.

Assessing value for money can be simply comparing like with like. When purchasing some goods this may be the case, but for the provision of services this is rarely the case. Earlier in this chapter, points to consider when assessing costs of services

Cost-effective services

have been mentioned. When assessing value for money it is important also to consider any capital expenditure required, along with the opportunity costs. Assessment of value for money for the purchase of goods and the supply of services cannot take place in isolation. The overall effects of changing or not changing working practices should be included.

Clinical goods and services

The assessment of value for money in clinical areas can be more complex. The delivery of effective health care depends increasingly on scientific and technological interventions which continue to develop at a rapid pace. Equipment can often be out of date almost as soon as it is installed. Assessment of value for money, therefore, can be difficult but is increasingly necessary. The purchase of new technological equipment often leads to an increase in its use which was not predicted. Simply having the equipment available leads to a decision to use it more often. With all interventions there are additional consumable costs which need to be included when assessment of the overall value for money is made.

The assessment of value for money for the purchase of equipment also needs to take account of the personal preferences of the users. An assessment of value for money should still be done even when there is a preferred product. This process is often achieved via an option appraisal exercise. This is another area where competitive tendering is used to good effect. If the suppliers of a product know they are in competition with other suppliers they must produce a competitive tender. If they are aware that they are likely to be the only supplier then the competitive edge is no longer there. Suppliers are there to make a sale and will offer 'deals' to persuade users to purchase their product and clinicians must always be aware of this. The standing orders of all NHS organisations will require the use of competitive tendering. A valid explanation of situations where this process has not been used must be provided. Assessment of value for money also needs to take account of the impact on other organisations. The impact of change on, for instance, social services departments as the result of earlier discharges must be assessed before action is taken. The decision may result in a more costly input for social services and this may still be the agreed outcome, because in overall terms it is the most effective outcome.

SUMMARY

The provision of cost-effective services depends on active management of the processes available to test services against best practice. Various options are available:

- Service reviews
- Service integration
- Benchmarking
- Market testing.

Whichever process is adopted it is more readily accepted as part of an ongoing process of continuous improvement. NHS organisations have a duty to provide value for money from the public monies allocated by ensuring resources are used wisely and well. They now also have a duty to ensure that the quality of services is acceptable.

The process of market testing should be project managed and should involve staff and their representatives at an early stage. The 'Best Value' approach linked to performance management processes in the NHS is likely to emphasise the need to involve users and concentrate on quality as well as cost.

References

Department of Health (1997) The new NHS: modern, dependable. London: The Stationery Office.

Department of Health (2000) The NHS Plan. London: The Stationery Office.

Cost-effective services

Application 8:1 *Eva Lambert*

Market testing – the process

In this account Eva Lambert describes the process of market testing. The NHS has guidelines laid down for this, but other organisations too have their protocols in order that a clear trail of accountability may be demonstrated. The European dimension is also to be considered. This is normally for services over a certain sum of money.

The process of market testing must be fair and rigorous. Ideally it should be managed as a project, with clear steps, timescales and agreed lines of authority and responsibility for the project team. All providers who are invited to tender must be dealt with fairly and consistently, via a process which is open and transparent.

Clearly, external providers will recognise that thel in-house provider has some advantages in knowing the service, whilst they will have the advantage of experience of differing forms of provision outside the public sector. The market testing procedure needs to include the steps listed in Box 8.1.1. Running alongside the process will be the determination of the in-house bid for the service. It is important that this is dealt with separately from the market testing process and that the staff involved are not those involved in the other aspects of the market testing process.

Staff involved in the process of market testing must ensure that the process is fairly tested, consulting relevant experts as appropriate. Typically, there are three teams of staff: a service specification team, an in-house tender team, and an evaluation team.

> **Box 8.1.1** Market testing: the steps
>
> - Drawing up the service specification
> - Advertising for interested providers
> - Evaluation of the providers
> - Invitation to tender from selected providers
> - Briefing of tenderers
> - Submission by due date of tenders
> - Evaluation of tenders
> - Presentation by shortlisted tenderers
> - Selection of successful tenderer
> - Award of contract
> - Commencement of new contracted service
> - Monitoring and review of service

DRAWING UP THE SERVICE SPECIFICATION

This process has been detailed in Chapter 8, using cleaning services as an example. The service specification team involved will usually include staff from:

- Relevant service
- Service users
- Supplies department
- Finance
- General management
- Personnel
- Staff representatives.

Wherever possible, staff involved in this stage should be different from those involved in the in-house team and the evaluation team.

The process is similar for any service, and requires that staff:

- determine the parameters of the service being tendered,
- detail exactly the service needed,
- consult with the end users of the service,
- determine any changes required, and
- finalise the specification.

It is important to ensure that this stage of the process is undertaken thoroughly, on the basis of this specification all the invited tenderers will detail the way they will provide the service and at what price. Often, tenderers are invited to visit the premises to see the current service and will be given opportunities to question the market testing team members but the tenders are submitted based on the specification details. If a service detail is not included the specification, then it will not be included in the tender.

ADVERTISING FOR INTERESTED TENDERERS

There are financial parameters laid down by the European Union. The intention to tender a particular service above a certain value must be advertised within the official journal of the European Community. A set period must then elapse for interested parties to notify their intention to tender.

EVALUATION OF POTENTIAL PROVIDERS

If there are a significant number of interested providers, then a process of evaluation takes place. This may be, for example, by an assessment of their ability to provide the service, consideration of the size of the organisation in relation to the size of the potential contract or their financial stability. If such an evaluation does take place then once again it must be fair to all interested parties and must stand up to scrutiny.

INVITATION TO TENDER BY SELECTED PROVIDERS

The agreed service specification, together with any necessary supporting documents must be sent to all potential tenderers. A return deadline is always specified. The invitation to tender usually requires a detailed cost analysis in a prescribed form to enable consistent evaluation with other tenders. On receipt of the detailed service specification some providers may decide not to proceed with the tender.

BRIEFING OF TENDERERS

In many cases the service required is large and/or complex and the opportunity is often provided for potential tenderers to meet a selected team to seek clarification of the requirements and to look around the premises. This briefing will include the in-house team members and in some cases it is the in-house expert who may be called upon to answer some of the questions. This may seem an excessive use of time, but it is important that all the tenderers receive the same information to ensure fairness of process.

SUBMISSION OF TENDERS

The invitation to tender will have included details of when and in what form tenders must be submitted. Once the date deadline has passed, the tenders will be opened formally in accordance with the relevant standing orders, and stamped, recorded and signed by the relevant officers.

EVALUATION OF TENDERS

The team involved in the evaluation of tenders will usually consist of some or all of the following:

- Professional expertise – often from another organisation
- Supplies department representatives
- Finance staff
- Service users
- Non-executive directors
- Personnel representatives.

Their task is to ensure that the various tenders are compared against the specification and against each other. This will involve:

- The financial details
- How they intend to meet the specification requirements
- How many staff they will use
- How many hours they will work
- At what productivity rate they will be expected to work

Market testing – the process

- How they will comply with relevant legislation, i.e. Health and Safety at Work
- How they will monitor compliance with standards
- What personnel policies they employ, e.g. for sickness and absence.

From this evaluation a short-list of potential providers will be made.

PRESENTATION BY SHORT-LISTED TENDERERS

This is an opportunity for tenderers to present themselves to the panel, and to elaborate on their written submission, highlighting their particular advantages. The in-house team will present their plans also and will be able to stress the factors of continuity and knowledge of the service. The panel will ask questions of the tenderers to clarify issues or to explore particular areas of concern. Although it can be a strange situation for in-house staff it is important that they present as serious tenderers.

SELECTION OF SUCCESSFUL TENDERER

When all presentations have been seen and evaluated the team must decide upon whom to recommend as the successful provider. Occasionally the outcome is clear and one tenderer has presented an outstanding tender, ahead of the others in price, quality, personnel and experience. More often there is more than one possible contender. The evaluation team must then debate the differences and agree on a recommended outcome. In some cases, and where the potential contract is neither large nor particularly sensitive, the team will have delegated authority to award the contract. In other cases the team must make a recommendation to the awarding authority.

AWARD OF THE CONTRACT

If the service has been tendered before and the outcome is not contentious, award may be as simple as approving a recommendation. This could be carried out by the senior management team, a senior officer or by the Board of the Trust or Health Authority. The authorised person or body will have been agreed at the outset either in line with the organisation's standing orders or, if appropriate, by agreement to waive the standing order. In all cases it is important that tenderers are informed of the outcome as soon as possible. This is particularly important where there is an in-house bid and where jobs are potentially at risk. Appropriate publicity of the event should be organised in order to communicate the outcome accurately and widely.

COMMENCEMENT OF THE CONTRACT

Irrespective of whether the contract is awarded in-house or externally, an acceptable commencement date must be agreed. If the award is to an external contractor then in-house relevant staff contracts will need to be terminated and/or transferred depending on the agreement. Service users will need to be informed and acquainted with the new personnel and appropriate monitoring arrangements implemented.

If the award is to the in-house team then it is likely that significant changes will have been agreed as part of the submission and these may require changes to staff contracts. The new budget for the service will be set at the contract value and any capital expenditure agreed as part of the award will be scheduled in the organisation's capital programme.

MONITORING AND REVIEW OF THE SERVICE

Monitoring arrangements for the service will have been determined as part of the market testing process. The monitoring will take the form of both service quality and price and results will be recorded and submitted as agreed. Contracts vary in their length but will normally have at least an annual review. Within the contract will be detailed terms of the procedures in the event of any failure by the contractor to meet the service specification. Depending on

Market testing – the process

the nature of the failure the contractor will be given time to correct the deficiency, but in extreme cases the contract may be terminated. Before the contract ends, arrangements for re-tendering the service or extending the contract will be agreed.

Delivering the business

Application 8:2   *Eva Lambert*

The human resource issues of market testing

This account follows on from Application 8.1 where Eva Lambert looked at the process of market testing. As has been said a number of times in this book, staff represent 70% of the NHS budget (and the biggest percentage of other health care providers budget too). People are unsettled by the prospect of change, and anything that can be done to support them to see change as an opportunity is both ethically, managerially and financially sound. What Lambert describes here is as much about change management as the management of resources.

The prospect of a service being market tested will almost always require change. The whole process of market testing is considered threatening for staff, as it may result in job losses. This is not always the case and normally depends on how well the service has progressed and kept pace with best practice. It is unlikely, however, that there will be no change, and most people find change threatening. Thus it is important to prepare staff well when services are to be reviewed, whether or not such a review includes a market testing exercise. Situations where service reviews are part of an ongoing process of continuous improvement within the quality framework of an organisation are likely to be accepted more readily than ad hoc reviews. It is important to involve staff in the process as early as possible. They should be encouraged to provide their own ideas on how the service could improve and discussion of these suggestions should be facilitated in an appropriate forum. The process of market testing will include clear documentation of what must be done and by what date (see Application 8.1). Human resource issues will be identified early in the process, ensuring adequate time for briefing staff and their representatives.

Whilst the staff of the reviewed service will be the main ones affected, care must be taken to ensure all interested and associated staff are kept informed. General communication of the process, timescale, people affected and briefing opportunities is essential. Many staff will benefit from having access to professional advice both from the personnel department and the local staff representatives.

INVOLVING STAFF REPRESENTATIVES

It is never too early to involve staff representatives in a service review, whether or not it includes market testing. They are appointed to ensure that staff interests are articulated and in most NHS organisations there will be regular meetings between management and staff representatives to provide time and opportunity for discussion. Staff representatives will try to ensure they obtain the best outcome for staff and initially they may oppose the market testing exercises, as they see the likely outcome as either job losses or less favourable terms for staff. If a market testing exercise is undertaken it almost always leads to changes in the way the service is provided and therefore the working practices of the staff employed. Early involvement of the staff representatives may slow the process down in the early stages but this has to be balanced against the benefits in longer term, both in terms of the outcome of the particular service review and in fostering good industrial relations.

It is unlikely that they will be involved in the formal assessment of the tenders. However ways should be sought to seek their views on areas of legitimate interest.

HANDLING CHANGES TO STAFF JOBS

The process of service reviews and market testing inevitably will lead to some changes which will affect the way staff work and therefore will have implications for their role and duties. The impact on staff may be minimal or it may involve re-profiling the workforce completely. In either case there must be an agreed process for handling the changes; this should be in line with the organisation's policies. It may be necessary to establish a dedicated team to interview every member of staff to explain what is happening and to acquaint them with the possible options open. It is essential that the organisation's policy for handling job losses is current and has been agreed with staff representatives before any market testing exercise starts. In most cases where job losses or major changes to jobs are required, the staff representatives will seek to avoid redundancy. It is often possible to achieve changes through natural wastage or retraining and redeployment of current staff. The option of redundancy is the last resort for employers, not just because it is an expensive option but because it is good employment practice to provide other opportunities for staff. The job losses/major changes policy of the organisation will determine how such changes are to be dealt with, including whether 'slotting in' of posts, preferential interviews, or competitive internal interviews, or competitive external interviews are to be undertaken.

DEALING WITH REDUNDANCY SITUATIONS

Any manager who is managing a service review needs access to professional personnel advice, particularly where major changes to jobs are expected. The personnel department will have expertise in industrial relations and will be familiar with the process for handling job losses. Employment legislation includes details of what action must be taken in a potential redundancy situation together with time limits when staff organisations and staff themselves must be informed. Their rights to redundancy payments will be governed by both their employment rights, the

The human resource issues of market testing

organisation's policies on redundancy and their rights under the terms of the NHS superannuation scheme (if they are a member). It is important that staff are given good advice and that they have sufficient time and help to consider their options.

Delivering the business

Chapter **Nine**

Quality in action

Michael J Cook

- • What part will clinical governance play in improving health care?
- • What is quality? Whose perspective?
- • Achieving the critical issues in quality improvement
- • Managing perceived service performance

- • The relationship of clinical governance to other quality management approaches
- • Planning for quality improvement
- • References

OVERVIEW

In Chapter 3 Brian Edwards considered the relationship between quality and policy. Here, Mike Cook takes this a stage further, and discusses the challenges and benefits of the implementation of quality processes. He looks at the management contribution via clinical governance and the national frameworks, and points out the key issue in it all: quality is here to stay, and it will be delivered as part of the service agenda. We are then taken through the history of the quality debate in the UK, and offered relevant theories.

There is no doubt that quality in health care is important and is receiving ever-increasing attention. This is being driven by current UK government policy and by increasing demand from consumers and pressure groups. The words used to describe quality initiatives may change but the drive for increased quality will be constant. No government will declare its commitment to reducing quality. In reality, more and more will be expected. For instance the British prime minister Tony Blair in September 1999 publicly stated that he wanted to see greater flexibility for patients: patients should receive treatment when it suits them, with the health care staff of their choice, in the health care facility of their choice. This raises public expectations, which in turn has an impact on those delivering the care.

This focus on quality in health care is not restricted to the UK. The same demands are being made across Europe and in America. Public promises are being made about increasing quality and the same is true in Australia. However, the financial support for health care, no matter how generous, will never be enough. Therefore it is vital that all money and resources directed towards health care are used as effectively and efficiently as possible. This is where a sound knowledge of management and of quality improvement becomes important.

Quality improvement in health care is gaining international attention, as a quick glance at the Quality in Health Care Journal confirms. England is no different. In England, a key document declaring a commitment to quality improvement was published in 1997, entitled 'The New NHS: Modern, Dependable' (Department of Health 1997). Sister documents have been published for Wales and Scotland and consultation documents in Northern Ireland (see Chapter 2).

In 'The New NHS, Modern, Dependable', the government sets out six important principles that underpin its vision of a modern and dependable health service fit for the twenty-first century – a national health service which offers people high-quality treatment and care, when and where they need it. The six important principles that guide the proposed changes are listed in Box 9.1.

Since 1997, many health care professional at all levels have been considering how these statements will be achieved. A new term to emerge in health care is 'clinical governance'. This has had a major impact on health care professionals. The most widely accepted definition of clinical governance is:

> Clinical Governance is a framework through which NHS organisations are accountable for continuously improving the quality

Delivering the business

Box 9.1   Six principles guiding changes to the NHS from 1997

1. Renew the NHS as a genuinely national service
2. Make the delivery of health care against new national standards a matter of local responsibility
3. Get the NHS to work in partnership
4. Improve efficiency so that every pound in the NHS is spent to maximise the care for patients
5. Shift the focus on to quality of care so that excellence is guaranteed to all patients
6. Rebuild public confidence in the NHS

of their services and safeguarding high standards of care by creating an environment in which excellence in quality of care will flourish.

Department of Health 1998a, p. 33

This definition is more complex than it first appears and is worth considering in more detail. The definition can be split into two parts. The first part ('Clinical Governance is a framework through which NHS organisations are accountable for continuously improving the quality of their services and safeguarding high standards of care') emphasises accountability and continuous improvement. The issues surrounding accountability have received a great deal of attention. One of the remarkable features is that clinical governance places accountability for quality directly and personally with the chief executive officer of the health care institution. It now seems surprising that this was not the case prior to the new legislation. This has shifted the attention of many chief executives away from the balance sheet and the accountants toward the clinicians and the care they provide. This seems to be a reversal of the trends in the early days of the internal market. The second part of the definition ('by creating an environment in which excellence in quality of care will flourish') has much wider and possibly more challenging implications. This will require a great deal of effort on the part of leaders in organisations.

An important health service circular (HSC/1999/033) provides the framework for quality improvement within the NHS (Department of Health 1999a). This framework, reproduced in Figure 9.1, describes the mechanisms whereby clear national English standards are being set through National Service Frameworks (NSFs) through the National Institute for Clinical Excellence (NICE). Local delivery of the service frameworks will be the responsibility of local clinicians who will be required to achieve high-quality health care provision. The Commission for Health Improvement (CHI) will monitor local delivery of the National Service Frameworks. Views of service users will be gained through a national patient and user survey. Clinical governance acts as the fulcrum around which quality improvement is achieved and monitored. These features will be underpinned by a modernised approach to professional self-regulation and extended lifelong learning for all clinicians.

The National Service Frameworks will:

- set national standards and define service models for a specific service or care group put in place to support implementation and
- establish performance measures against which progress within an agreed timescale will be measured.

It is interesting to consider the direction of the arrows in Figure. 9.1, in particular the arrow coming down from NICE to clinical governance, with no reciprocal upward arrow. This in some ways may be an oversight, as it is important that wherever possible clinicians get involved in influencing this powerful group. Failure to do so will lead to a bias in the decision-making framework towards a central government-controlled agenda. This may not be in the best interests of care in the wider context. Some care groups may be excluded; indeed it is interesting to see

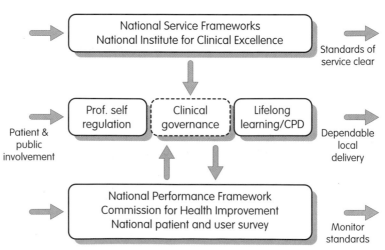

Figure 9.1 Framework for quality improvement within the NHS.

that older people are starting to feel marginalised with respect to health care equity.

WHAT PART WILL CLINICAL GOVERNANCE PLAY IN IMPROVING HEALTH CARE?

Bush (1994) refers to governance as the exercise of public authority to achieve commonly agreed goals that are determined by a democratic majority. Important in this definition and related to the concept of clinical governance is the notion of democratic majority and subsequent power. In other words, to achieve clinical governance will mean a major shift in thinking in the NHS. Clinicians now have the opportunity to address the possibility of domination by particular groups and others with greater influence in health care. However, with this opportunity for clinicians comes the responsibility to achieve meaningful change for patients. It is anticipated that clinical governance will increase staff accountability and responsibility, and therefore enhance empowerment.

According to Bernreuter (1993), clinical governance provides a method of increasing control over practice by increasing and formalising staff participation in the system. Other definitions exist but, common to all definitions, is the tenet of individual professional accountability and interdependent collegial responsibility for decision making. If grasped, this can place real power in the hands of the professionals. Clinical governance is more than about reshaping the formal organisational structure. It requires a change in philosophy and attitudes that requires careful consideration. Clinical governance is in part a reflection of a greater global change. We are moving from an Industrial Age to a Chip Age, where the interconnectedness of actions and outcomes are becoming better understood. This is outlined in Box 9.2.

Box 9.2 Comparison of the Industrial Age and the Chip Age

Industrial age	*Chip age*
Linear thinking	Systems thinking
Compartmentalise	Indistinct boundaries
Process orientated	Outcome orientated
Fixed job requirements	Fluid work requirements
Predictable impacts	Variable impacts

Quality in action

There is nothing magical about governance and the shared decision making philosophy that will underpin its success, but it has the potential to transform the way things are done. However, it must be recognised that clinical governance requires a radical change in thinking and not merely tinkering at the edges by drawing new organisational charts. It is about autonomy to innovate in clinical settings, not just about fiscal accountability. It needs clinical staff to be provided with an environment where they have the confidence and support to pursue an opportunity and prove what can be done, not what would be done if certain issues were resolved (e.g. increased staffing, more money or better working conditions). It is about working with what is at a particular point in time. This is where investment in staff by management is vital.

One approach is to involve staff more in workplace activity by delegating appropriate tasks. However, staff need to know what level of decision making they are being delegated, and the authority they have. All too often groups have a task delegated without a clear remit, and often without knowing how far they can go. It is useful to think of allocating levels of decision making when delegating activity. For instance, level 1 can be data collection and reporting back to the manager, level 2 may be data collection and making a recommendation, and so on, until a level is reached where full decision making is delegated, including the authority to spend a certain amount of money.

Quality is a concept that is here to stay, so it is important to work with it so that you can become its masters not its slave.

WHAT IS QUALITY? WHOSE PERSPECTIVE?

So what is quality? It means different things to different people, thus a clear shared understanding has been difficult to achieve. Everyone has a general understanding of quality. It describes how individuals value particular aspects of a service or product that they are considering. Definitions abound: 'quality can ... be defined as what the customer states it is' (Wiggans & Turner 1991, p. 183); 'Quality in public service can be defined as fully meeting customer requirements at the lowest cost' (Øvretveit 1992, p. 2). Others define quality in terms of features of the service, for example accessibility, relevance to need equity, social acceptability, efficiency and effectiveness (Maxwell 1984). This definition makes an important point: it is not only important to

(Delivering the business)

produce satisfaction for those health care 'customers' who receive the service, but also to ensure access for all those that need the service. It is important to include, alongside the patient's judgments of the service, a professional definition of need, and a professional judgement of the extent to which a service meets the patients' needs.

However, even this reference to need becomes complex as patients may not know what they need, or may ask for treatments that may be inappropriate or harmful. Boothe (1990, p. 67) maintains that 'quality relates to customers' perceptions, not the perceptions of those who provide the service.' Therefore, the provider must gain an understanding of the perceived needs of the customer. It is also important to determine who these customers are. A wide definition of customer is required and this includes staff working in the organisation, employers, patients, health authority purchasers, NHS Executive bodies and health service providers. To be successful, it is important to understand how quality is being defined by all relevant organisations.

ACHIEVING THE CRITICAL ISSUES IN QUALITY IMPROVEMENT

If an institution is to engage meaningfully in quality improvement activities then it must know how people perceive their service. This can form a valuable baseline from which to measure future changes. Peters & Waterman (1982) and Walker (1990) identify that listening to customers is a priority for those wishing to make customer service effective.

Three factors are a good starting point for organisations when attempting to work with others to improve quality:

1. *Willingness to discuss and negotiate*   Managers have to be able to share with staff their views and to listen to other viewpoints. Very clear ideas as to what is to be achieved are essential.
2. *Meeting and understanding needs*   Different sections or groups will have different perspectives. This means that managers must know how to reach consensus decisions so that all parties can sign up to the changes required.
3. *Quality of the staff*   This is perhaps the most vital factor. An effective manager must know what strengths particular staff bring. In addition, the manager must know something of the working interactions between group members. This

Quality in action

means getting involved, being able to negotiate and find ways of getting staff talking and listening to each other and their viewpoints.

These are crucial perspectives to be considered by the manager before embarking on a particular quality improvement route.

Simply putting a system in place for customers to air their views is not sufficient. Moores (1991) pointed out that a wide gulf often exists between customer expectations and what companies believe these expectations to be. He went on to claim that customer-driven companies go to extraordinary lengths to ensure a harmonisation of these two sets of perceptions. Peters & Waterman (1982) gave many examples of senior managers of companies such as Digital, McDonald's and Hewlett-Packard, spending significant periods of their time 'in the field', undertaking sales roles, cleaning and staffing car parks.

In the NHS this means people at all levels becoming aware of what others do in the organisation. This can be achieved by shadowing others and especially those whom one would not normally work alongside, or by developing a forum for sharing views on a regular basis. This is easy to suggest, but difficult to achieve in the NHS where workloads are increasing and the luxury of time to shadow is difficult to find among the many other pressures facing clinicians. However, it is not impossible to achieve and may well prove more valuable than more conventional classroom-based learning activity. Often an 'outside' view can provide almost immediate improvement (Box 9.3).

Whilst the purchaser views are important, is it also important to gain the views of consumers, i.e. those who use the service or products. 'Knowing what customers expect is the first and possibly most critical step in delivering service quality' (Zeithmal et al 1990, p. 51). The problem with the intangible nature of

---

Box 9.3 Example illustrating the impact of an 'outside' view

The nursing staff in an American hospital was experiencing an increase in drug administration errors. In this hospital it was routine for drugs prescribed by medical staff to be re-written by nursing staff onto a nurse dispensation sheet. Using a common business quality improvement technique called Pareto analysis, an outside observer quickly spotted that it was possible to trace most of the errors to this re-writing. The nursing staff had not considered this as a source, but the outside observer was able to identify it after spending only a short time in the area.

health care, from the perspective of both provider and user, is that customers 'don't know what they are getting until they don't get it' (Levitt 1981). In other words, not all customers can tell the provider all their requirements before the service provision commences. It is necessary then for the provider to put in place mechanisms for eliciting the views of customers before and during the period of service provision.

It will be interesting to see the impact of the planned NHS user surveys. By undertaking such surveys expectations will be raised that action will be taken on the findings. This may become an additional source of pressure on the NHS towards further quality improvement.

MANAGING PERCEIVED SERVICE PERFORMANCE

A key factor that influences customers' perceptions of service performance is reliability. This involves consistency of performance and dependability, specifically performing the service at the designated time, and providing the required service safely and competently. A distinctive aspect of services is that customers are often part of the production and delivery processes, the quality of the service provided will be influenced by the customers' input. It is therefore possible to include customers as organisational members or 'partial employees', and to attempt to influence their behaviour through the process of organisational socialisation. This may include setting out patients' responsibilities or service user guides. Indeed, occasionally consideration is given to very tangible responsibilities to patients, in the form of charges for non-attendance at outpatient clinics. This would no doubt have a negative impact on the views of the NHS, and may hit hard those that can least afford such an imposition. More positive aspects could indicate the shared responsibilities between client and carer, such as self-medication. In the longer term this may generate a very positive customer loyalty impact.

It can be seen, therefore, that quality improvement is a term that describes a continuous process of developing the product or service provided. Indeed, this is the whole essence of the government document 'A First Class Service' (Department of Health 1998a). To achieve this requires both staff and organisational development, which is clearly articulated in the human resource White Paper 'Working Together: Securing a Quality Workforce for the NHS' (Department of Health 1998b). It can be

Quality in action

seen that quality is the fulcrum that enables an organisation to build on existing strengths and good practices, and it enables staff to use new methods in a systematic way to improve quality and to resolve quality problems.

This focus on staff interactions and relations is a central point of many successful quality programmes and is as important as introducing new systems, specifications and measurements. Walker (1990) believed that even if a product or service itself does not meet expectations, excellent personal service can redeem the situation. He showed that a formal system for assessing the strengths of staff is necessary to maintain the highest standards of personal service, and isolated three aspects central to such a system (Box 9.4).

Jackson (1992) reiterated these points by offering a guiding principle of getting people to measure their work for its value to the customer, rather than its cost to the company. Similarly, Asher (1990) believed that the only way to identify what the customers want is to 'see it through their eyes'. If health care is to continue to improve then it is vital that clinicians and health care managers learn to see the service through the eyes of the user. With clinical pathways this is becoming possible. Such a fundamental review of service provision provides an ideal opportunity to seek user views. Very often some of the most obvious improvements cost very little in monetary terms but do require staff to rethink some ingrained approaches to work.

There needs to be as much emphasis on changing people's attitude towards their work, as on training them to use specific tools and techniques. Tools are only used if people want to use them, and they are only used properly if people have been

---

Box 9.4 Three aspects central to an assessment of staff qualities

1. *Skills and knowledge* Lack of these is immediately offputting to customers. This can then result in a lack of confidence both in the organisation and by the individual delivering the service, leading in turn to increasingly poor service.
2. *Attitudes* The employee must be motivated to perform their tasks to a consistently high standard. While definition of attitudes is often complex, the behaviours resulting from good attitudes are often easy to observe.
3. *People systems* These include such activities as recruitment and selection, induction, training, appraisal, promotion, incentives, and facilities and equipment.

Delivering the business

trained to use them and have the time to do so. It is the role of leadership to ensure that mechanisms are in place to support staff in their quality improvement activities. Leadership is pivotal in quality improvement and must not be neglected, a point emphasised by Juran (1989) and Deming (1986), who identify that 80–94% of organisational problems are leader created. As quality improvement activities are designed to reduce an organisation's problems then leaders must accept responsibility for this. This is emphasised clearly in the NHS nursing and midwifery and health visiting strategy 'Making a Difference' (Department of Health 1999b). However, what seems to be absent is an outline of the type of leadership that is required. Effective leaders work with very different approaches, from the autocratic to the truly inspirational. Employers in health care need to decide which they wish to employ.

THE RELATIONSHIP OF CLINICAL GOVERNANCE TO OTHER QUALITY MANAGEMENT APPROACHES

A close examination of clinical governance in comparison with other quality improvement approaches reveals many similarities. Management commitment, measure for progress, explicit and shared values, operating in defined teams, effective staff development and the needs of customers all feature widely. Review becomes the norm, and common to both clinical governance and other quality management approaches is the involvement of staff to bring about change. This requires a major re-think of people's roles and responsibilities in health care. For clinical governance to be successful it is vital that all staff at all levels become involved in shaping the service. The assumptions that certain professionals will lead aspects of provision have to be challenged and re-thought. This may make for an uncomfortable period for service providers and perhaps even service users. But if this challenge is taken up meaningfully then the longer term outlook will be positive.

A key point to recognise is that quality management approaches require a decentralised management style. Can this be achieved in the health service? According to Girvin (1996), a strong hierarchical centralised management approach has pervaded, and certainly the general approach of this administration appears to be one of central command and control. Indeed, the implementation of CHI, NICE and NSFs which embody an ethos of strong central control may, in the longer

259

term, be counter-productive. To prevent this local staff must be able to influence local delivery directly. This means getting involved and aware of what is being discussed centrally.

Clinical governance will not be sufficient by itself to deal with the pace of change required. Dahlgaard et al (1997) emphasise this point in their research on leadership and quality improvement. They identified that the ability of the leaders and success of the organisation are strongly correlated, a view reinforced by Joiner (1994), who states that effective leadership will be a deciding factor in which organisations survive in the twenty-first century.

Senge (1990), when describing his work on a computer model with insurance personnel, states that in most cases the groups he worked with dealt quickly with the problems posed to meet short-term goals. However, they failed to look in the right places to see the long-term consequences of their action. It is this ability to look in the right place that leaders and managers must learn to develop if organisations in which people work are going to succeed. For example, if one is trying to develop a new approach to care then it is important to involve all stakeholders implicated in the change. If one considers the prescribing incident described in Box 9.3, identifying the problem was relatively easy, but making the changes to ingrained practice was probably less than easy. Medical staff who for years had relied on nursing staff to interpret their sometimes vague instructions were frustrated that they had to write precisely and carefully. Pharmacy staff had trouble interpreting medical staff writing when ordering drugs. This may suggest that the root cause of the problem lay with the medical staff, however some nursing staff contributed to the problem because they resented the perceived loss of power of losing their own medication charts. Whilst the change was made with the best of intentions to save nursing time and reduce errors, the hidden implications were not revealed as staff impacted by the change were not involved in the decision making process.

PLANNING FOR QUALITY IMPROVEMENT

Planning is not merely the simple process of determining the inputs, controlling the processes and measuring the outputs. The process is more complex. Strategies often emerge from patterns. These patterns emerge as work is being done and people find ways of solving problems, often by means of experimentation. This happens because it is not always possible to anticipate

Delivering the business

everything. Most organisations operate within a mix of intended and emerging strategies. Leaders need to recognise this process and help people to discard inappropriate emergent strategies whilst nurturing potentially good ones. The skill is to spot which to nurture and which to end. A further important skill is to end the inappropriate strategies sensitively.

In designing a quality improvement strategy, asking specific questions before setting out on this major initiative is vital for success. As a starting point, Parker (1993) identified some important questions: Why are we dissatisfied with what we have got now? What is wrong with it? What could we be like? For example, using the medication example:

- Why are medication errors increasing? What is going wrong? How can this situation be improved? How are medications prescribed and supplied to patients?
- What goes wrong? Can we identify route causes?
- How would a solution look? Can we eliminate all errors? Are we willing to work together to improve this situation?

By reviewing these points, it is possible to focus upon the vital issues within the change process.

Having decided that there is a requirement for a quality improvement activity, the following principles, based on the work of Flood (1993) are essential to consider:

- Management must lead, and engender a 'no blame' culture
- Customer requirements must be agreed
- Customer/supplier relationships should be understood and improved
- Who does what needs to be ascertained. What does the supply chain look like?
- Once a new system is in place, it is important to aim for no errors
- Continuous improvement is the goal
- Management must measure for success
- It is important to do the right things and do things right first time
- More effective communication is essential
- Training is essential
- It should be agreed in advance how staff will be recognised for success
- Successful involvement must be recognised and praise given.

The work of Deming (cited by the Department of Trade and Industry 1991) reinforced and synthesised the work of the quality gurus within his system of 'profound knowledge'. He combined the common features to create four interrelated factors: theory of systems, theory of statistics, theory of knowledge and theory of people.

- *Systems* are processes that underpin quality, and emphasis is placed on the need for leaders to understand the relationships between functions and activities.
- *Statistics* refers to the importance of measurement of quality standards. This includes knowledge about variation, process capability, and control charts, interactions and loss function. In order to accomplish effective quality improvement these must be understood. It is the manager's role to share and make available statistical data and trends about the service. For instance, using the example of administering medication, to collect numbers of errors over a set period of time, and the types of those errors would be a simple but meaningful data set.
- *Knowledge* implies all plans require prediction based on experience; an example of success cannot be effectively copied unless the theory is understood.
- *People* requires the psychological needs of people to be met, and relates closely to the work of Peters (1989) and Handy (1994), who emphasise the importance of recognising individuals within organisations.

To complete the strategic quality design process it is essential to consider customers, employees, competition and key business processes. This enables the organisation to establish goals that are aligned throughout all its parts. It is not possible to give a rigid format that can be adopted by all organisations. The method used must depend on the culture, structure, systems and internal and external pressures being faced at the time of introduction. All these factors determine the effectiveness of the quality process and thus whether it achieves the agreed goals.

Quality strategies used to develop the internal environment of an organisation in readiness for quality improvement activities focus upon maximising its strengths, while recognising and minimising any weaknesses. In quality terms, 'the culture of an organisation is arguably the most important component of the internal environment' (Wiggans & Turner 1991, p. 183).

Culture is a perspective, it is the way things are viewed within organisations. It is the core of an organisation's philosophy of 'how things are done'. The culture of the business affects everyone in it, and everyone who comes into contact with it. It affects the lives of everyone who depends upon it. A culture conducive to quality improvement must be nurtured. This is a key management role and relies heavily upon active management participation. Managers need to have access to in-depth knowledge of the operational features of a business activity or to have access to staff who do have this knowledge. Without this, decisions are taken in a vacuum of ignorance. A characteristic activity of the effective manager is 'management by walking about' (MBWA). Operationally, this means making time to visit and be involved at the sharp end of care.

Wiggans & Turner (1991) state that managers embarking on a quality improvement route need to:

- gain their own managers' commitment,
- involve the workforce,
- know how to motivate staff,
- give people more responsibility for their own activities, and
- set and agree measurements for improvement.

and this can only be achieved in a blame-free culture. These are key factors in the process of organisational development and thus, implicitly, quality improvement. A collegial, interdependent way of working to achieve quality in the workplace must become the norm – no longer can the responsibility be focused on one person, 'the quality advisor', as once occurred. Quality is everyone's business, and everyone's responsibility. Leaders must recognise and be prepared to harness the collective skills of others in the goal of continuous improvement. Quality improvement takes energy, commitment and passion. Quality champions must be identified and supported. The pay-off can be an improved organisation with an enhanced reputation, reduced costs and increased satisfaction of customers, staff, contractors and an increasingly positive environment for people to work in.

References

Asher J M (1990) Quantifying quality in service industries. Total Quality Management 1: 89–94.

Bernreuter M (1993) The other side of shared governance. Journal of Nursing Adminstration 23(10): 12–14.

Boothe R (1990) Who defines quality in service industries? Quality Progress February: 65–67.

Bush T (1994) Theories of education management, 2nd edn. London: Paul Chapman.

Dahlgaard J J, Larsen H Z, Norgaard A (1997) Leadership profiles in quality management. Total Quality Management 8(2&3): 516–530.

Quality in action

Department of Health (1997) The new NHS: modern, dependable. London: The Stationery Office.

Department of Health (1998a) A first class service: quality in the new NHS. London: The Stationery Office.

Department of Health (1998b) Working together: securing a quality workforce for the new NHS. London: Department of Health.

Department of Health (1999a) HSC/1999/033. A first class service: quality in the new NHS. Feedback on consultations. London: Department of Health.

Department of Health (1999b) Making a difference: strengthening the nursing, midwifery and health visiting contribution to health and healthcare. London: Department of Health.

Department of Trade and Industry (1991) The quality gurus. London: DTI.

Deming W E (1986) Out of the crisis. Cambridge, Massachusetts: MIT Centre for Advanced Engineering Study.

Flood R L (1993) Beyond TQM. London: John Wiley & Sons.

Girvin J (1996) Leadership and nursing: part one history and politics. Nursing Management 3(1): 10–12.

Handy C (1994) The empty raincoat: making sense of the future. London: Hutchinson.

Jackson D (1992) The art and science of service. Marketing Business 12: 23–31.

Joiner B L (1994) Fourth generation management: the new business consciousness. New York: McGraw-Hill.

Juran J M (1989) Juran on planning for quality. New York: Free Press.

Levitt T (1981) Marketing intangible products and product intangibles. Harvard Business Review May–June: 94–102.

Maxwell R J (1984) Quality assessment in health. British Medical Journal 288(1): 470–471.

Moores B (1991) Lessons from some of the USA's most respected service providers. Total Quality Management 2: 269–277.

Øvretveit J (1992) Health service quality: an introduction to quality methods for health services. London: Blackwell Scientific.

Parker K (1993) TQM: just another far eastern package deal? Works Management December: 22–25.

Peters T (1989) Thriving on chaos: handbook for a management revolution. London: Pan Books.

Peters T J, Waterman R H (1982) In search of excellence. New York: Harper & Row.

Senge P (1990) The fifth discipline: the art & practice of the learning organization. London: Doubleday.

Walker D (1990) Customer first – a strategy for quality service. Aldershot: Gower.

Wiggans T, Turner G (1991) Breaking down the walls. Total Quality Management 3 (3): 183–186.

Zeithmal V A, Parasuraman A, Berry L L (1990) Delivering service quality: balancing customer perceptions and expectation. New York: Free Press.

Delivering the business

Risk management – in support of quality

In this application, Julie Hyde links the process of risk management with the overall drive towards quality. She points out that active risk management, both clinical and non-clinical, is a relatively new concept for many in the NHS, and that all costs which result from poor risk management must be met from within the organisational budget, resulting in significant lost opportunity costs. In addition, the cost of insurance premiums aimed at transferring financial risk must also be met from the organisation's own budget.

The term 'clinical governance' emerged as a result of the publication of the English White Paper 'The New NHS: Modern, Dependable' (Department of Health 1997), and subsequent papers, most particularly 'A First Class Service: Quality in the New NHS' (Department of Health 1998). The two key elements within clinical governance are the notions of quality improvement and financial accountability.

All NHS organisations are required to have in position robust processes for managing clinical governance, and with effect from April 2000, the chief executive officer of each Trust is required to sign an assurance statement, on behalf of the Board, about quality, in addition to the annual report. Trusts tackled the requirements to put management processes in position in different ways, but all have designated responsibility for clinical governance to a senior person, usually either the nurse or doctor member of the Board.

Initially, the assumption was that this was a new concept – clinical governance workshops, conferences and publications offered support and ideas to those charged with its implementation. At the same time, huge change initiatives were happening in the NHS, including the formation of Primary Care Groups (PCGs) and Primary Care Trusts (PCTs) in England, Local Health Care Cooperatives (LHCCs) in Scotland and Local Health Groups (LHGs) in Wales, which were only part of the devolution agenda for health. Throughout the UK, Trusts have been merging and 'downsizing', resulting in upheaval both in organisational workload, and for the staff. Once again, many staff were required to apply for their own jobs, often competing with colleagues they had worked with for many years.

As people started to investigate further the concept of clinical governance, it became apparent that whilst the statutory requirement and the CEO personal responsibility may be new, the component parts of clinical governance were not. Clinical governance was only new in that it strengthened and formalised the framework within which to deliver processes and activities which were well established.

Clinical governance is about quality, and it requires a comprehensive quality improvement programme, with built-in processes for monitoring and evaluating care. This is not a new idea as such, but now the framework is formalised and more robust. There is a requirement that wherever possible evidence-based interventions will be used, and these incorporated within a range of national standards. This requirement will be monitored and supported by the National Institute for Clinical Excellence (NICE) in England and Wales. This has the organisational status of a Special Health Authority and is independent in its activity. In Scotland, the equivalent of NICE is the Scottish Health Technology Assessment Centre (SHTAC), and this body too has Special Health Authority status. In Northern Ireland, as yet no formal bodies are established, but the principles of clinical governance are accepted.

A key element of clinical governance is the management of risk, and the drive for quality has brought this activity to the top of the government agenda. As society in general becomes more litigious, it comes as no surprise that the number of claims in the system is increasing. It is estimated that there may be in the NHS as much as £1 billion of outstanding liabilities in cases of clinical negligence. The cost of litigation continues to rise, and thus is a real issue for managers and clinicians alike, as any claims must be met from within the financial envelope of the Trust's budget. Clearly defined policies to manage both clinical and non-clinical risk are mandatory.

Risk management programmes normally progress through three stages:

1. Identifying the risk
2. Analysing the risk
3. Controlling the risk.

These processes are well established in industry and the private sector, but in relative terms are new to the NHS. Up until April 1991, all NHS properties had Crown Immunity, and thus the responsibility for risk was less focused. To some extent this is reflected in the attitudes of some NHS staff – they have had to learn to be more attuned to the proactive process of risk management. This may be in relation to something as simple as not leaving chairs in front of firedoors, or to a more complex clinical issue.

The effective and focused management of risk is the responsibility of all, and is an active way of contributing to the quality of the patient experience. Most organisations have a designated risk manager in post, but it is important that all staff understand the three-stage process in order that they can contribute to a coherent programme of risk management within the organisation.

THE THREE-STAGE PROCESS OF RISK MANAGEMENT

Identifying the risk

This is a data-gathering exercise aimed at establishing the kinds of risks which may occur within the organisation, and to make judgements about how often these are likely to occur. It is important that all pieces of data and information are accounted for, as analysis of many serious incidents has shown that ostensibly small issues can combine to cause a serious mishap. Complaints are a useful source of material, particularly if a theme is recurrent.

Risk management – in support of quality

Analysing the risk

This is a complex process, which involves a clear understanding of the risks identified, and examining them within a framework of incidence, causes and impact. A range of management tools such as flowcharts, pathway charts and cause and effect diagrams are useful processes with which to analyse the material gathered.

Controlling the risk

This involves introducing a range of focused activities which may include physical safety features (e.g. handrails), or organisational controls in the form of a range of protocols or guidelines. It is important that the whole process of risk management is done in a measured way; kneejerk, overreactive interventions are not likely to be as effective as carefully thought out, reasoned decisions.

The second phase of controlling the risk is to decide whether the Trust will retain the responsibility for the risk, i.e. will it deal with the consequences (including financial responsibility) of any mishaps, or will it seek to transfer the risk to some form of insurance. Up until the introduction of the internal market which resulted in Trusts having the legal status of a business, it was impossible to insure against any risk. Thus the option to transfer risk via insurance has only been possible (for first wave Trusts) since April 1991. As in any insurance negotiation, the cost of the premium will mirror the risks.

References

Department of Health (1997) The new NHS: modern, dependable. London: The Stationery Office.

Department of Health (1998) A first class service: quality in the new NHS. London: Department of Health.

Section **Three**

THE ADDED VALUE OF COLLABORATION

Partnerships and collaborative working are high on the agenda of government today, both at an organisational level and at the level of the individual practitioner. Chapter 10 offers a selection of examples of how partnerships can work in a range of different contexts.

In Chapter 11 Christa Paxton explains how to get the best out of partnerships with the voluntary sector, and includes a directory of useful addresses, and Gill Poole demonstrates the benefits to all of genuine collaborative working between different groups of people.

Chapter **Ten**

The importance of partnership

OVERVIEW

PART 1: THE INDEPENDENT SECTOR IN CONTINUING CARE (LINDA NAZARKO)

The nursing home sector continues to play an important part in the delivery of health care. As the elderly population grows, and as people live longer, the demand for care will increase. The need for the NHS and the independent sector to work in partnership has never been greater. The development of this relationship means that the 'boundaries' between the acute sector in the NHS and the independent sector can become less rigid, allowing older people to move more easily between sectors as their clinical need dictates. As Jill Ellison writes in Application 4.3, the independent sector has an important part to play in enabling the NHS to make best use of its acute services. Increasingly nursing homes can offer complex packages of care, and often an older person would prefer to stay in their own environment, rather than be admitted to an acute hospital ward. This is more likely to happen if specialised services from the NHS can be provided within the nursing homes as part of a partnership agreement.

Most people think of nursing homes as small, individual organisations, but few are aware of the size of the nursing home sector. Nursing and dual registered homes employ 276 000 people and care for 275 000 residents (Laing 2000). Nursing home staff serve 426 000 meals per day and launder 852 000 kg of laundry per week. Employee salaries total £2.516 billion every year and nursing homes contribute £6.291 billion annually to the national economy.

The average nursing home employs 41 staff and spends £390 000 a year on salaries. A quarter of all registered nurses now work in the independent sector (UKCC 1997). The number of nursing home staff studying part-time is 11 774, equivalent to the annual intake in a small university. Nursing homes are now the major providers of continuing care (Department of Health 1997a).

The role of independent sector homes

At their inception, nursing homes aimed to care for people who would no longer benefit from active medical treatment. Now the nursing home sector cares for a wide range of people with diverse care needs. In the USA, a quarter of all people admitted to nursing homes are discharged home after a period of rehabilitation. In the UK, most people admitted to nursing homes are admitted for permanent care. Researchers in the UK (Millard et al 1995, Nazarko 1997) suggest that older people in the UK could benefit from similar rehabilitation programmes. The Royal Commission

The added value of collaboration

on Long Term Care published in March 1999 acknowledges the value and contribution of rehabilitation programmes, and has recommended the development of a national strategy.

Many older people wish to remain at home and their carers wish to care for them at home. However, caring for a frail older person at home is extremely demanding. A large number of nursing homes now offer respite care to enable carers to have a break, thus enabling them to continue the caring role for longer. A number of people enter nursing homes in the later stages of dying and require highly skilled palliative care. Many nursing homes are now developing specialist dementia services to meet the needs of this client group.

Since the publication of 'The New NHS: Modern, Dependable' (Department of Health 1997b) the focus of care has shifted further towards the community setting. As Primary Care Groups (PCGs) focus on the needs of the local population, nursing homes are taking a key role in providing appropriate care for older people, in partnership with other agencies.

Purchasers of nursing home care

Currently, nursing homes cater for three distinct groups of purchasers:

1. Social services departments
2. Self-funding individuals
3. Health Authorities.

The number of people funding their own care has fallen steadily since 1995. There are several possible explanations for this. Older people are now more aware that nursing home care is means tested. Some older people may be giving away their assets to avoid having to pay for nursing home care. Older people living in nursing homes are the only client group who have had their access to nursing care means tested. In response to criticism, the government has increased the eligibility thresholds. In 1990, an older person with savings above £3000 was unable to obtain state funding to meet the costs of nursing home care; now the threshold is £16 000, and many more people are able to claim state funding. In 1998, Laing suggested that 75% of people cared for are state funded (Laing 1998a,b).

Self-funding individuals meet all the costs of their nursing home care from their own purse. Health Authorities have a legal responsibility to draw up and publish their eligibility criteria for NHS care and this varies from area to area. In some areas, the

Health Authority assumes responsibility for funding the care of older people who are terminally ill and have a life expectancy of 6 months, in other areas it is 6 weeks and in others 2 weeks. Reports (CSAG 1997; Haskin & Patel 1998) criticise this situation as inequitable and urge the introduction of national eligibility criteria.

The challenges facing nursing homes

In less than 10 years, nursing homes have moved from the margins of continuing care to the mainstream. Nursing homes face major challenges in their efforts to deliver high-quality care, some of which are outlined in Box 10.1.

Current regulations focus on quantitative measures such as the size of a room, the number of staff, and the number of shared rooms, as these are easy to quantify. The quality of nursing care is much more difficult to measure, and nursing home staff share those challenges with other professionals.

Expectations within the sector are rising in line with society in general as resources fall in real terms. New National Required Standards, which all nursing and residential homes must meet, are being introduced by government. It is anticipated that some small homes may have difficulty meeting these standards for a number of reasons and may be forced to leave the market.

Appropriate assessment of need is the key to providing quality care in any environment. Current assessment protocols may fail to recognise the nursing needs of older people (Bugner 1996, CSAG 1997, Haskin & Patel 1998), and increased shared working across the independent sector and the NHS aims to enhance understanding of nursing needs in different contexts of care.

In recent years, the independent sector has moved from being a minor player to the major provider of continuing care and standards within the sector have risen enormously. People

---

Box 10.1   Challenges faced by nursing homes

- Regulations and a payment system determined by a medical model
- Rising expectations from relatives, regulators and residents
- Tensions between health and 'social care'
- Resources that are falling in real terms
- Difficulty recruiting and retaining registered nurses

The added value of collaboration

moving to nursing homes increasingly expect to be offered a single room with en suite facilities. Many homes offer a choice of lounges and dining areas, and facilities such as craft rooms, snoozelen rooms and hydrotherapy pools once considered a luxury are becoming more common.

As the percentage of older people in society increases, the need to provide transparent and seamless care increases. This can be best achieved in partnership with the full range of health and social care providers.

PART 2: COMMUNITY HEALTH COUNCILS (ANGELINE BURKE)

Community Health Councils have an increasingly important part to play in health care today. They represent the spirit of openness in government, and foster partnerships and shared responsibility across all stakeholders. Note that although at the time of writing this chapter is correct, the NHS plan 'A Plan for Investment. A Plan for Reform' presented to Parliament in July 2000, proposes the abolition of CHCs in England by March 2002. The proposals are subject to approval by Parliament.

Community Health Councils (CHCs) were established in 1974 as statutory, independent bodies to represent the interests of the public in the NHS. A number of scandals had emerged in long-stay hospitals and it became clear that statutory bodies could not manage hospitals and represent patients without a potential for conflict of interest. As a result, CHCs were created and have a statutory right to:

- be consulted by the health authority on changes in the NHS,
- enter and inspect NHS premises,
- receive information from the NHS,
- have formal meetings with the Health Authority, and
- receive comments from the Health Authority on the annual report, which CHCs have a duty to publish.

There are 204 Community Health Councils in England and Wales with similar bodies in Scotland and Northern Ireland. Each CHC is run by a paid staff, usually the equivalent of two or three full-time workers, and in addition, normally there are between 16 and 30 members who work on a voluntary basis. The members come from the local community and are nominated by

The importance of partnership

the local authority (half), elected by the local voluntary sector (one third) and appointed by the regional offices of the NHS Executive or the National Assembly for Wales (one sixth). Members should be committed to the National Health Service and should bring to the CHC expertise and experience which will help the CHC carry out its functions. Members are expected to abide by the 'Code of Conduct for CHC Members' when carrying out their work with respect to the CHC (Department of Health 1995). Research has shown that CHC members spend between 8 and 20 hours per week on work connected with the CHC (Arnold et al 1995).

CHCs have to fulfil certain duties as laid down by the Regulations, but beyond those duties they are autonomous and thus have developed in different ways over the years. It has been suggested (Buckland et al 1994) that there are five 'types' of CHCs:

- Independent challengers
- Health authority partners
- Independent arbiters
- Patient's friends
- Consumer advocates.

CHCs tend to demonstrate features from all of these 'types' at some stage during the course of their work (ACHCEW 1996a). Autonomy has its advantages. For example, it allows and encourages innovative practice. On the other hand, the lack of uniformity amongst CHCs has, from time to time, led to criticism, as the standard of service may differ between CHCs across the country. Some criticisms may be justified but others should be considered in terms of the very limited resources that CHCs have to work with (ACHCEW 1997). The current level of resources for CHCs is less than 0.1% of the total NHS budget. In response to some of the criticism, CHCs are working together to develop a set of performance standards.

Working with individuals and the community

CHCs are able to offer impartial advice and assistance to individuals and local groups. Although it is not an explicit statutory requirement, much of the work of CHCs involves assisting and supporting people who wish to make a complaint about the services and treatment they have received from the NHS. It has been estimated that in 1995 the total number of complaints handled by CHCs was in the region of 20 000 (ACHCEW 1996b). Some CHCs also encourage people to help themselves by, for example, providing or assisting with the development of advocacy services.

Working with health professionals and others

Although CHCs have no explicit statutory remit concerning primary care, many CHCs have forged links with local practitioners. CHCs are frequently asked to help general practitioners to establish patient participation groups and to carry out patient satisfaction surveys. CHCs are also able to advise GPs on how to involve patients in setting standards.

CHCs must meet in public at least once every 3 months. Many meet every month and take the opportunity to invite health professionals to attend the meetings either to discuss specific initiatives and developments such as proposed cuts in family planning services, or simply to talk to members and the public about their specific jobs and the role that they play within the Health Authority or Trust.

When exercising their right to visit NHS premises, CHCs take the opportunity not only to talk to patients but to talk to staff at all levels. It is useful to talk to staff because CHCs can get their personal, perhaps 'unofficial' views, as well as the 'official' views of the establishment. Following a visit to NHS premises a CHC will prepare a report of the visit which will include any necessary points for action. The management will then be given the opportunity to comment on the report.

The statutory remit of CHCs does not cover local authorities. However, because of developments in care in the community and the need for health and local authorities to work in collaboration, some CHCs have taken the opportunity to establish links with local authorities. These are mainly with social services departments but sometimes involve other departments such as housing and environmental health, in recognition of the potential impact that these areas have on the health of individuals.

In an ever-changing NHS, health care watchdog groups, who work in the interests of the public and patients and to represent their views to the policy-makers, are necessary now more than ever. Despite the fact that many people are unaware of CHCs, or have heard about them but are unclear about their role 'CHCs do have a record of effectiveness and now need new powers and resources to meet new challenges' (ACHCEW 1997, p. 55).

The importance of partnership

PART 3: NHS AND PRIVATE CARE – A SHARED APPROACH (ROS GRAY)

As more and more people take out private health insurance, either as individuals or as part of their employment package, many more of the public have experienced both private and NHS health care. Increasingly over recent years, and particularly as a result of the internal market of the 1990s, both sectors have pooled their knowledge and resources in a genuine attempt to make best use of resources for the majority of the population.

You have seen earlier in this book the way the political agenda in the UK influences the delivery of health care, and its influence on the interface between private and NHS care is no exception. The debate of pragmatism of resource utilisation versus ideology continues. However, 'The NHS Plan' published in 2000 makes explicit reference to the desirability of the public and private sectors collaborating.

Communication between private and public sectors

A number of options is available to people who need clinical treatment. Most people use the services of the NHS automatically, even though some of them have purchased private medical insurance. Others take an initial private consultation in order to be seen more quickly and then choose to use the NHS for the treatment prescribed. The remainder choose to use an independent provider for their health care needs either by using private medical insurance or paying for the service themselves.

Whichever approach people use, there needs to be effective channels of communication between both sectors of health care to ensure that all patients receive the best treatment, that duplication of effort is avoided and that precious resources are not wasted. There is evidence of this willingness to share, an example being the use of independent sector facilities by the NHS to reduce waiting lists. This makes use of available resources in the independent sector, where the average occupancy for independent sector hospitals is approximately 60%, in contrast to the NHS which at times supports occupancy levels of 120%. The sharing of equipment, notes, results and X-rays as both sectors try to meet client requirements is appropriate and ensures that no information about the patient is lost.

Quality of care improvement

Patients expect and deserve a high-quality standard of care whether they are cared for within the public or private sectors of health care and new quality initiatives in the NHS are aimed at ensuring quality of care in both sectors. Health care professionals from all disciplines work in both sectors: many consultants have NHS practices and private practices and nurses may supplement their income by working extra shifts in a different sector. In addition, there are a number of examples where specialist practitioner expertise has been purchased or jointly funded to cover a particular client caseload that includes patients from both the NHS and the independent sector. Clearly it is unacceptable for professionals to apply different principles and standards of care in different environments. Patients in the NHS and the independent sector locally share the same consultant pool and to develop separate pathways of care for the same client group would represent a waste of resources.

As the National Institute for Clinical Excellence (NICE) becomes established and evidence-based practice emerges as the norm, delivered within a framework of clinical governance, quality of care should improve. Whilst NICE targets NHS care provision, the independent sector is committed to working within the same quality parameters, and this initiative offers opportunities for joint working.

One of the biggest areas of growth using a shared resource is the employment of breast care specialist nurses. The private insurers as purchasers of health care in the independent sector have been quick to follow the lead of the NHS in cancer care. Cancer services represent in excess of £80 million of benefit spend for a large insurer, so to target this area of care makes sense not only from the human perspective, but also from an economic one. Many independent hospitals, however, do not have enough patients to support investment in a specialist service such as breast care. As a result many have developed a joint appointment and a true partnership that maintains quality of service demonstrated by better clinical outcomes.

Although cancer services, where the standards being applied have been widely acknowledged and accepted by clinicians for some time, is a good place to start, the principle will not be easy to adopt in other disciplines. Often there is debate about the efficacy of treatments and limited scientific evidence to support one treatment option over another.

The importance of partnership

Lifelong learning – a shared responsibility

A further concept outlined in 'The New NHS: Modern, Dependable' (Department of Health 1997b) is the principle of lifelong learning. As professionals work increasingly across blurred boundaries of private and public health care, the commitment to develop a workforce that is fit to deliver quality health care in the future is a shared responsibility. Increasingly, providers in the independent sector provide work-based placements, where students experience the differences in health care provision and are able to apply their knowledge to the whole spectrum of health care in the UK. This is to be welcomed, as historically there has been criticism aimed at the independent sector for not contributing directly to education programmes for pre-registration studies.

PART 4: INTERFACES AND RELATIONSHIPS WITH VOLUNTARY AGENCIES (MARGARET GOOSE)

The voluntary agencies have a tremendously important part to play in health care in the UK. At their heart is the principle of partnerships, both with the client groups and with the statutory services. Further detail about the voluntary sector can be found in Chapter 9.

The voluntary sector is complex and wide-ranging in its activities, containing a large number of different types and sizes of organisations; there is no typical voluntary sector organisation. The Deakin Report on the Commission on the Future of the Voluntary Sector (Deakin 1996) states that one uniform feature is the concept of independence and a key factor is the presence of volunteers: 'the life-blood of the sector'.

The term voluntary agency is not synonymous with charity because the Charity Commission registration is determined by other criteria, including public benefit, no distribution of profits, no involvement in party politics and the trustees administering charities act voluntarily and without personal benefit.

There are over 188 450 registered charities whose combined annual income is over £19.7 billion, £12 billion of which comes via fundraising; 70% have income of £10 000 or less per annum and 271 have annual incomes in excess of £10 million. Only

The added value of collaboration

30 000 have any paid staff at all, 6000 with five or more, and over 100 with 1000 plus.

Handy (1998) suggests that there are three broad categories of organisation within the voluntary sector:

- mutual support, such as Alcoholics Anonymous and Gingerbread,
- service delivery, such as Barnardos and Action Aid, and
- campaigning, such as Greenpeace.

Many organisations fall into more than one category; for example, Shelter both campaigns for homeless people and also provides its clients with advice and housing.

The health field

The voluntary sector in the health field is similarly wide-ranging in its activities and size. There are 170 organisations listed under 'The Health College' of the National Council for Voluntary Organisations (Box 10.2). Some are concerned with a single

---

Box 10.2 National Council for Voluntary Organisations: Members

2 Care
ACT
Action for Dysphasic Adults
Action for Sick Children
Action for Victims of Medical Accidents
ACTIONAID
Age Exchange Theatre Trust
AIDS Care, Education and Training
Alcohol Concern
Alcoholics Anonymous
Arbours Association Ltd
Arthrogryposis Group
ASSERT
Association for Continence Advice
Association for Spinal Injury Research and Reintegration Rehabilitation
Association of Youth with Myalgic Encephalo-Myelitis
Breast Cancer Campaign
Breast Cancer Care
British Colostomy Association
British Dental Health Foundation

The importance of partnership

Box 10.2 Cont'd

British Diabetic Association
British Epilepsy Association
British Institute for Brain-Injured Children
British Lung Foundation
British Lymphology Society
British National Temperance League
British Performing Arts Medicine Trust
British Red Cross Society
British Thyroid Foundation
British Tinnitus Association
British Voice Association
Broadreach House
Brook Advisory Centres
Cancer and Leukaemia in Childhood
Cancer Black Care
CancerBACUP
Cancerlink
Cardiomyopathy Association
Changing Faces
Child Psychotherapy Trust (The)
Children's Head Injury Trust
Climb
Community Health UK
Community Housing and Therapy
Continence Foundation (The)
Crossroads – Caring for Carers
CRUSAID
Cruse Bereavement Care
Depression Alliance
Depressives Anonymous
Disability Alliance Educational and Research Association
Disabled Living Foundation
Down's Syndrome Association
Dyspraxia Foundation
Dystonia Society
Eating Disorders Association
Ectopic Pregnancy Trust
Enuresis Resource and Information Centre
Ex-Services Mental Welfare Society
Exercise England
Federation of Multiple Sclerosis Therapy Centres
Field Lane Foundation
Fortune Centre of Riding Therapy
Forum of Chairmen of Independent Hospices
Foundation of Nursing Studies

The added value of collaboration

Box 10.2 Cont'd

Gardening for Disabled Trust
Guillain Barré Syndrome Support Group of UK
Haemophilia Society
Hamlet Trust
Headway National Head Injuries Association Ltd
Health Quality Service
Hearing Concern
Help the Hospices
Homoeopathic Trust
Hope UK
Huntington's Disease Association
ia – The Ileostomy and Internal Pouch Support Group
IBS Network
Immune Development Trust
Incontact
Institute for Complementary Medicine
Institute for the Study of Drug Dependence
Intensive Care National Audit and Research Centre
International Alliance of Patients' Organisations
Inward House Projects Ltd
ISSUE
Judith Trust (The)
Kings Medical Research Trust
Leprosy Mission (The)
Leukaemia Care Society (The)
London Lighthouse
Long-Term Medical Conditions Alliance
Lupus UK
Lymphoma Association
Macfarlane Trust
Macmillan Cancer Relief
Manic Depression Fellowship
Marie Curie Cancer Care
ME Association
Medic-Alert Foundation
Medical Foundation for the Care of Victims of Torture
Ménière's Society
Mental After Care Association
Migraine Trust
MIND
Miscarriage Association
Motor Neurone Disease Association
National AIDS Trust
National Association for Patient Participation
National Association for the Relief of Paget's Disease

The importance of partnership

Box 10.2 Cont'd

National Asthma Campaign
National Cancer Alliance
National Council for Hospice and Special Palliative Care
National Eczema Society
National Federation of Spiritual Healers
National Federation of the Blind of the UK
National Meningitis Trust
National Pyramid Trust (The)
National Schizophrenia Fellowship
National Sports Medicine Institute of the UK
NHS Confederation
No Smoking Day
Obsessive Action
Pain Concern UK
Patients' Association
Philadelphia Association
Phoenix House
Pituitary Foundation
POPAN
Prader–Willi Syndrome Association (UK)
Prostate Cancer Charity
Psoriatic Arthropathy Alliance
QUIT
Reach
React
Retinoblastoma Society
Rett Syndrome Association UK
Revolving Doors Agency
Richmond Fellowship
Ronald McDonald House
Royal College of Nursing
Royal Society for the Prevention of Accidents
Royal Society of Health
Ryde Inshore Rescue
Samaritans (The)
SHE Trust (Simply Holistic Endometriosis)
Sickle Cell Society
Sir Robert Mond Memorial Trust
Society for Endocrinology
Society for Mucopolysaccharide Diseases
St John Ambulance
STEPS
Stroke Association (The)
Survivors of Bereavement by Suicide
Tacade

Box 10.2 Cont'd

Teaching Aids at Low Cost
Terrence Higgins Trust
Thrive
Tourette Syndrome (UK) Association
Turning Point
UK Brain Tumour Society
UK Coalition of People Living with HIV and Aids
UK Public Health Association
United Response
Urostomy Association
Vision Homes Association
Visyon
Vitiligo Society (The)
Walsingham Community Homes
Women's Nationwide Cancer Control Campaign
Women's Therapy Centre
Womens Health
Young Minds

disease, providing information, advice and mutual support (e.g. Breast Cancer Care), others deliver services (e.g. The Richmond Fellowship), concentrate on campaigning (e.g. ASH), or fund medical and other health research. A few combine all four aspects (e.g. The Stroke Association) and some are national only (e.g. The Patients' Association) or have local branches, some of which operate independently (e.g. MIND).

Source of funds

There is no one source of funds; some voluntary organisations rely mainly on government or other grants, some receive money from the statutory sector, most will fundraise through membership subscriptions, donations, legacies and trusts as well as selling goods and services. Annual reports will give a breakdown of income and expenditure.

Change of relationship

The independence of the voluntary sector is guarded jealously by its members, staff and volunteers. In health and social services, voluntary organisations have frequently undertaken pioneering work which has subsequently proven its value and

The importance of partnership

285

been adopted by the statutory services as good practice (e.g. Age Concern's support for patients on discharge from hospital, and many areas of children's services piloted by Save the Children Fund). Some of this type of work was funded by grants, some undertaken by professionally qualified staff, and much has been supported by trained volunteers acting in locum familias (e.g. Samaritans).

With tightening financial regimes in the public sector, those organisations which historically received grants from the Department of Health, NHS Authorities or Social Services Committees increasingly found it necessary to justify the effectiveness of their work. With the introduction of the internal market philosophy following the NHS and Community Care Act 1990, the contract culture led to funds being allocated for services delivered to a specification. Many voluntary organisations were concerned at this fundamental shift, not because explicit quality standards were being set for the first time, but because their independence was threatened: the funder could now determine what service should be given, by whom and in what way.

Voluntary organisations had always competed for grants but the contract culture produced more overt competition with the private sector and greater insecurity of income from statutory services who had previously also contributed towards infrastructure costs as well as lobbying and advocacy activities. This, coupled with general changes in society and in patterns of care, has led to some voluntary organisations altering the nature of their services.

Interfaces with statutory health care

Some voluntary organisations, such as the WRVS and Leagues of Friends, have worked in hospitals for many years, running shops, teabars and patients' libraries as well as fundraising for patients' amenities and equipment. More generally, the partnerships with statutory health care operate at all levels:

- National:
  campaigning
  research
- Local:
  provision of services to groups
  involvement in planning of services and influencing change

Individual:

working with individual patients and their carers.

Health professionals increasingly have found themselves working with people from voluntary organisations, for example in self-help groups and as advocates.

The consumer movement is gaining ground in health care as in other walks of life. Voluntary organisations frequently provide specialist information and advice to patients and the public, which will help them to help themselves, assess the services provided and challenge health professionals.

The White Paper 'The New NHS: Modern, Dependable', published in December 1997, emphasises the need for collaboration, partnerships and alliances rather than competition (Department of Health 1997b). In Health Action Zones, voluntary organisations are mentioned specifically as key players. The flexibility of most voluntary organisations to adapt to changing circumstances would suggest that they can, once again, pioneer different ways of meeting need in health and social services.

Nationally, the government announced in January 1998 an arrangement between itself, voluntary organisations and the statutory sector which guarantees the independence of the voluntary sector. Leaders of voluntary organisations are generally sceptical of political rhetoric but will seize every opportunity to ensure that voluntary organisations continue to play a significant role in British society.

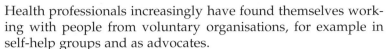

PART 5: MANAGING THE WORKPLACE AS A LEARNING ENVIRONMENT (JOHN HUDSON)

Initial education and training and continuous professional development has always had a place in the life of the health care professional. However, this emphasis has become greater over the past few years as a number of professional groups have made more explicit the requirement to remain fit for practice. Whilst it is important to remember that continuous professional development is not just about engaging in formal education programmes, clearly the relationships and attitudes towards learning as a continuous and expected process in every facet of the professional experience is the key to ensuring that the public has the services of a flexible, committed workforce.

The period since 1970 has seen a major increase in the amount of time and attention devoted to the more effective management of human resources. This has been accompanied by a growing acknowledgement amongst employers from all sectors of the importance of investing substantially in the professional and personal development of their workforce. Even in the public service sector, such investment is not entirely motivated by altruism. Staff who feel their employer is interested in their personal fulfilment and who are supported to undertake the professional development necessary to advance their career as well as meeting increasing employer expectations, will be better motivated, more committed, and thus happier and more effective in their work.

This has occurred against a background of general change in society at large, characterised by a move away from the dramatic emphasis once placed on learning as an activity largely completed during the first two decades of life, towards a concept of lifelong learning. The culture shift has been driven by the need to prepare individuals for the continuous adaptation to changing circumstances which will undoubtedly characterise their future working life wherever they are employed.

Both these trends have brought learning into the workplace as a normal activity as never before, thus creating new challenges for managers, and none more so than in the health care sector. Long used to training they now are increasingly becoming involved in education, with all that this involves. As an integral part of their role managers must now see themselves in partnership with their staff as learners, and with universities, as more formal providers and accreditors of higher education. As a consequence they must now manage the workplaces for which they are responsible as learning environments which in turn influences the quality of the patient/client experience. This link between lifelong learning and quality in the NHS is made explicit in the White Paper 'The New NHS: Modern, Dependable' (Department of Health 1997b) and the subsequent consultation paper 'A First Class Service' (Department of Health 1998). Learning, especially professional development, has now become much more explicitly a shared responsibility between the individual, his/her employer and the education provider. This calls for new kinds of partnership, a joint commitment to the learning agenda, a shared understanding of the objectives and outcomes of learning and the establishment and maintenance of excellent functional relationships between the partners in the triad.

As with any partnership, the individual members each have their own agenda, and progress comes through first recognising this and moving on to agree the common purpose which brings them together. In the management of education and training for health care professionals, this common purpose can be summarised as the desire to produce a practitioner fit for practice, fit for purpose and fit for award.

Fitness for practice refers to the ability of a practitioner to satisfy at least the minimum standards of practice laid down by the appropriate (national) regulatory or licensing body to ensure the safety of the public at large, and thus be awarded a licence to practise. Fitness for purpose is the ability to carry out professional practice in the work setting to the standards demanded by an employer, often set out in the core of a job description. Fitness for award requires that the prospective practitioner has achieved the academic criteria required by the end of a formalised accredited programme of learning. Clearly, whilst each of these three requirements will be the primary focus of concern for different members of the partnership, all three must be achieved to meet the common purpose.

Meeting the challenge

First, learning in the workplace must be legitimised by managers. There must be an explicit valuing of learning activities, along with a clear expectation that staff should constantly engage in them. Health care managers may perceive a conflict between their explicit core purpose of providing clinical services to patients and clients, and the provision of learning opportunities for students and practitioners. Although self-evidently true, it is usually not helpful to point out that without such learning opportunities there will be no future practitioners and therefore no health care services! The more effective management strategy is to ensure, by close collaboration with university providers that learning activities are structured in such a way as to be an integral part of service delivery, thus creating a culture of continuous learning. A work-based project can be a particularly useful tool here. In addition to being an effective learning vehicle, a well-planned and structured project can produce valuable outcomes in the workplace.

Secondly, managers need to develop effective relationships with the higher education sector and its academics. The commissioning arrangements for health care education have given

The importance of partnership

managers excellent opportunities through the education purchasing consortia to exert a much more direct influence on the content of curricula, and on the ways in which they are delivered. However, these new arrangements recognise quite explicitly that education and training for health care professionals is a joint responsibility between the university sector and the service itself, and so lay great emphasis on the importance of long-term developmental relationships. To ensure that these relationships are effective, and to deliver on their own objectives, managers of the business of health care must participate fully in the management of learning. This should be across the whole structure of liaison with higher education, from strategic advisory boards through to curriculum development and programme monitoring teams. Managers need to be proactive in articulating clearly to the higher education sector the learning needs of their staff, and in working with them in the planning and implementation of joint programmes which deliver 'the three fitnesses'. Equally importantly, they will need to collaborate with universities to put in place suitable processes for the careful monitoring of the outcomes of learning to ensure its continuing relevance to the needs of staff and the requirements of the workplace, with appropriate feedback systems.

Education and training for health care professionals is a major investment in this country, and vital to the continued delivery of a high quality health service. The NHS alone spends around £1.4 billion annually through its consortia on non-medical (i.e. all professions except doctors and dentists) education. The staffing crisis of the late 1990s, rolling over into the twenty-first century, serves as a stark warning of the potential consequences of failing to manage this huge investment well. The effective deployment of such an enormous and important resource must be a high priority for any health care manager.

References

Arnold C, Etherington P, Taylor B (1995) Community Health Councils at the millennium: 'the views of CHC members'. London: ACHCEW.

ACHCEW (Association of Community Health Councils for England and Wales) (1996a) Handbook for CHC members. London: ACHCEW.

ACHCEW (Association of Community Health Councils for England and Wales) (1996b) An analysis of the complaints work of CHCs. London: ACHCEW.

ACHCEW (Association of Community Health Councils for England and Wales) (1997) CHCs making a difference. London: ACHCEW.

The added value of collaboration

Buckland S, Lupton C, Moon G (1994) An evaluation of the role and impact of Community Health Councils. Southsea: University of Portsmouth.

Bugner T (1996) The regulation and inspection of social services. London: Department of Health & Welsh Office.

CSAG (Clinical Standards Advisory Group) Chaired by Professor Dame June Clark (1997) Community health care for elderly people. London: The Stationery Office.

Deakin N (1996) Meeting the challenge of change: voluntary action into the 21st century. The report of the commission on the future of the voluntary sector. London: NCVO.

Department of Health (1997a) Statistical Bulletin 97/26. Community care statistics 1997: Residential personal social services for adults, England. London: The Stationery Office.

Department of Health (1997b) The new NHS: modern, dependable. London: The Stationery Office.

Department of Health (1998) A first class service: quality in the new NHS. London: The Stationery Office.

Department of Health, Welsh Office. NHS Cymru Wales and NHS Executive (1995) Code of conduct for Community Health Council members. London: Department of Health.

Handy C (1998) Understanding voluntary organisations. London: Penguin.

Haskin C, Patel C (1998) Review – long term care. Better regulation task force. London: Cabinet Office.

Laing W (1998a) A fair price for care? Disparity between market rates and state funding of residential care. York: York Publishing Services.

Laing W (1998b) Care of elderly people market survey, 11th edn. London: Laing & Buisson.

Laing W (2000) Care of elderly people. Market survey, 13th edn. London: Laing & Buisson.

Millard P, Smith E, Bennett M (1995) The right person? The right time? The right place? An audit of the appropriateness of nursing home placements post Community Care Act. Commissioned by SELHCA. Published internally by St George's Hospital, London.

Nazarko L (1997) Getting better? The quality of care in UK nursing homes. Unpublished MSc dissertation, South Bank University, London.

Royal Commission (1999) With respect to old age long term care – rights and responsibilities. A report by the Royal Commission on long term care. London: The Stationery Office.

UKCC (1997) No nurses working in independent sector. London: UKCC.

The importance of partnership

291

Application 10:1   *Marilyn Ekers*

Continuing care policy

The introduction of the continuing care policy has been a challenging one in all areas of the country. This application details a real case study of processes put into place to ensure a seamless, equitable service for those people in Leeds who need continuing care. The key issue here is the need and value of partnership working. At the time of the introduction of the continuing care guidance the requirement to work in partnership with other agencies was less well accepted, and this case study represents a model of good practice both in terms of policy application and partnership working.

In February 1995 the Department of Health published guidance requiring Health Authorities to review their arrangements for, and funding of, continuing health care. The outcome of that review would be a local policy and eligibility criteria to determine who would get continuing care services funded by the NHS.

The requirement for such a policy largely arose because of the view that the NHS had withdrawn too far from commissioning and providing continuing care: it was not providing the full spectrum of care. In particular, the NHS had closed long-stay geriatric hospitals or wards and older people were, instead, placed in nursing or residential homes mainly in the private sector. Consequently, local authorities (social services) felt they were bearing costs which should have been the responsibility of the NHS.

There was also growing political and public concern that because health care is free and social care is means tested, any shift from health care to social care meant that people

The added value of collaboration

could be paying for care which they had expected to be free.

The issue came to a head when the Health Service Commissioner (Ombudsman) published a report about a case in Leeds. The complaint involved a man whose family was required to pay his nursing home fees following discharge from hospital. The Ombudsman felt that because of his condition, the man should have received fully funded NHS continuing care.

THE POLICY

The Department of Health's requirement was that Health Authorities should develop local policies and eligibility criteria for continuing health care, consult on them and publish a final version by 1 April 1996. Consultation would have to include full involvement of local authorities, all GPs, NHS and independent sector providers and representatives of users and carers.

Coverage

The policy was to be wide-ranging, to cover:

- older people, including those with mental illness,
- people with dementia,
- younger adults requiring continuing health care as a result of illness or accidents, and
- children.

It was equally wide-ranging in its coverage of services, going beyond continuing inpatient care to include:

- specialist medical and nursing assessment,
- rehabilitation and recovery,
- palliative health care,
- respite health care,
- community health services,
- specialist health support to people in residential care or the community,
- primary health care, and
- specialist transport.

Continuing care policy

Key issues to resolve

- How to make a political judgment about withstanding the pressure to invest in beds against the desire to invest in community health services.
- How to manage the development of the policy and eligibility criteria.
- Which stakeholders to involve and at what stage.
- How to deal with the range of client groups and services in one policy.
- How to engage with users, carers and the general public in a meaningful way on a very complex and sensitive issue.
- How to re-invest in services in a managed way to reflect health care needs.
- How to gain the agreement of the local authority, the key stakeholder, to the policy and eligibility criteria.

Local context in which the policy was being developed

- That the local NHS had withdrawn too far from continuing health care (e.g. there were no NHS continuing care beds for older people).
- That there was overemphasis on acute health services.
- That there was relatively poor investment in community health services.
- That there was no new money from the government attached to the introduction of the policy.
- That there was intense scrutiny (national and local) of the development of the policy and eligibility criteria because of the particular local circumstances.

APPROACH TO DEVELOPING THE POLICY

In view of the importance attached to the introduction of a continuing care policy and the intense interest aroused, significant resources were allocated to its development. A project management approach was adopted to ensure the required product was achieved within the deadline laid down. The project team comprised a project manager (full-time) with a senior team drawn from within the Health

The added value of collaboration

Authority, comprising public health medicine, finance, nursing and primary care. The team was led by an executive director of the Health Authority. The fact that general management and other professionals were working together on these political, clinical and financial issues was seen as essential if all the implications of the policy were to be realised. To sustain this level of resource to the project over a long period required the commitment of the highest level of the Authority.

In the early stages of the project whole days were set aside each month away from the office to ensure the team could work uninterrupted. Some of the time was thinking time, some of it was time devoted to collecting and analysing information and some of it was reflective time which prepared the negotiators for their role.

The project was mapped in terms of activities, timescales and lead responsibilities to make the best use of individuals' time outside of the project. Every meeting was minuted with action points so that progress could be clearly monitored and reviewed and to ensure that all team members were clear about the tasks and their own responsibilities. It was a robust process that provided building blocks for development. The project team tasks and output are outlined in Table 10.1.1.

Table 10.1.1 The tasks/project plan

Project team tasks	Output
Define the project	Description of project
Agree definitions	Shared understanding and glossary
Define current baseline	Assessment of demand
Prioritise areas to define new eligibility criteria	Agreed criteria and priority areas
Determine consultation process	Mechanism agreed by management team
	Process agreed with partner agencies
Determine implementation process	Proposals agreed by management team
Determine monitoring and evaluation arrangements	Draft document for consultation
Write policy document and eligibility criteria	
Consultation	Respond to written comments and make presentations
Revise policy and criteria in light of comments received	Final policy and eligibility criteria published

Continuing care policy

In parallel to this process, a small group of local consultants were invited to advise and comment on the Health Authority's emerging criteria. The consultants represented all the specialties and client groups to be covered by the new policy.

NEGOTIATION WITH THE LOCAL AUTHORITY

Once the project team had been established and its work defined, an invitation was extended to the local authority to form a joint project team. This team would aim to ensure congruence between the Health Authority's eligibility criteria and the local authority's eligibility criteria for nursing home and residential home care. It was essential that the local authority was not presented with a 'fait accompli' and so needed to be involved in the development stage of the work.

After each meeting, the agreements reached were minuted by an exchange of letters so that there could be no misunderstandings later. These letters also acted as a record of progress.

The discussions with the local authority needed to identify the authority's particular concerns and priorities. The Health Authority needed to find the key issue on which the local authority's support would hinge. It had always been of great concern to the local authority that community health services were underprovided and that their services had been used to fill gaps. Emphasis was therefore placed on this by the Health Authority in drawing up its investment plans as part of the policy. It was deemed essential that the Health Authority's commitment to its policy was shown by publishing its investment intentions for continuing health care in the policy document.

CONSULTATION

In order to meet the requirements of HSG(95)8 and to ensure a wide understanding and debate, a draft policy statement was drawn up for consultation. The period of consultation lasted 3 months and included:

The added value of collaboration

- Circulation to a wide range of organisations and individuals in Leeds, including the Community Health Council (CHC), Local Authority, Citizens Advice Bureau, local MPs, NHS Trusts, the Local Medical Committee (LMC) and the NHS Executive.
- Presentations to the LMC and GP fundholders, voluntary organisations, CHC, groups of GPs and consultants, Trust managers.

A significant challenge was how we should consult with service users, carers and the public in general. The judgement was made that it would not be possible to have meaningful dialogue on such a complex issue in structured public meetings. Instead, a market research company was commissioned to recruit a number of focus groups. Some groups were very specific, such as carers of people with dementia or young disabled people; others were cross-sections of the public. As well as the Health Authority gaining valuable information, these focus groups had an unforeseen by-product: for many of the carers and older people attending it was a rare opportunity to leave home and mix with other people in a relaxed setting as substitute carers and transport were provided to enable them to participate. Many said how much they had enjoyed the sessions.

IMPLEMENTATION

Practical issues

The first key issue in implementation was how to ensure staff in the local Trusts and social services were aware of, and understood, the new policy and eligibility criteria. They would be the people interpreting and applying them. A series of open, daytime meetings were held at the local Trusts at which the policy and eligibility criteria were presented by senior managers from the Health Authority and social services. These sessions took place around the time the policy was to come into operation. Clearly, not all staff would attend these sessions so a summary document was prepared and made widely available throughout the agencies.

A booklet for service users and carers was produced, briefly explaining the policy and how to access the new

Continuing care policy

297

independent review procedures for continuing care. A strong attempt was made to write the booklet in plain English and to make it freely available in hospitals. The local and national experience has been a very low referral rate to the process. It is not clear why this is so.

Monitoring

Clearly, although the policy and criteria had been agreed and information disseminated to staff, there would be issues arising during the early implementation period which had not been foreseen. It was also essential that the Health Authority had a good understanding of the impact of the new policy. For these reasons, the project team continued to meet but less frequently to consider how emerging issues should be addressed.

Resolving problems

The project manager's role continued on a full-time basis to deal with the many ad hoc queries that came in by telephone and letter, and to meet on a regular basis both NHS provider and local authority colleagues to discuss and resolve problems. The Health Authority had requested each local Trust, and the neighbouring ones, to nominate a lead person for continuing care with whom we could communicate.

Some of the problems posed were an obvious direct result of the new policy. In particular, determining the respective responsibilities of the Health Authority and local authority for purchasing the care of people who needed a high level of health and social care which was to be jointly commissioned. Clarification on terms used in the criteria, such as 'specialist nurse' or 'technical feeding' was also a frequent question.

What was not expected was the volume of queries about what should happen to people who did not meet the criteria under the policy but still required health care. Another significant issue was the number of referrals of people who needed specialist health equipment on discharge from hospital, especially expensive pressure-relieving mattresses. The demand for this equipment rose dramatically.

The added value of collaboration

Two approaches were needed to deal with those challenges: first, by the project manager being the point of contact for queries and being able to respond immediately to requests for guidance and clarification, and secondly, by categorising the issues and developing longer term strategies to deal with them.

On the question of 'who pays for what?', the Health Authority appointed a case manager to negotiate directly with the local authority and independent sector providers to agree funding and ensure appropriate placements were made for long-term care. For equipment, a review of the loan equipment service was commissioned and a new purchasing policy adopted for patients being discharged to nursing homes. In conjunction with the local community health service provider, a revised protocol for assessing for pressure-relieving equipment was drawn up and a tissue viability nurse post funded.

CONCLUSION

Two years on, the original policy and eligibility criteria are still in place. Some of the issues that arose in the early days have disappeared or been resolved by specific action. However, new challenges continue to arise and continue to be dealt with in the same ways. Some learning points are listed in Box 10.1.1.

Box 10.1.1. Joint working: learning points from developing the policy

- Involve your partner(s) at an early stage.
- Be clear about your joint objectives and the approach to achieving them.
- Record all agreements.
- Share information and provide evidence for your assumptions.
- Regularly review progress and take action accordingly.
- Listen!
- Identify one or two of your partner's key priorities that you can address.
- Keep talking.

Continuing care policy

Application 10:2   *Martin Shreeve*

Working together

This case study outlines a process in partnership working between three groups to improve services for older people.

THE NEED FOR A SHARED VISION

The implementation of the NHS and Community Care Act in 1990 brought new challenges into the system for practitioners and managers in the fields of nursing, care of the elderly medicine, and social care. The need to respond to increased demand and public expectation within a tightly restrained resource skin can lead, and had in the past led, to cost shunting and a blame culture. Representatives from the British Geriatric Society, the Royal College of Nursing and the Association of Directors of Social Services, who shared a common commitment to improving services for older people and a concern for the tensions in the system, decided to act.

DIVIDED BY A COMMON LANGUAGE

Drawn together to consider NHS guidance on continuing care, representatives of the three organisations recognised that services for older people would improve if a whole system approach was taken. Patients' needs would be best met if all the resources in the system were used to optimum effect. Before a shared vision can be developed, however, a common understanding is required. We soon found that whilst our values and overall objectives often corresponded, the language we used sometimes got in the way. Were we talking about patients, clients, consumers, service users or customers? Is it 'the elderly', 'older people' or 'senior citizens'? These were the relatively easy questions to answer. More complex concepts such as rehabilitation or assessment were often interpreted quite differently by the different organisations. Each organisation carried values about practice and territory, the skills required and, often, who had primary responsibility.

WRESTLING WITH A COMPROMISE

Whilst acknowledging competition for resources existed between the organisations, there was an overriding recognition that more could be achieved by working together to a common goal. The goal was easy insofar as everyone shared a common commitment to improving services for older people within a macro system that often failed to see senior citizens as a priority. By putting the older person at the centre of the system, then examining the roles of the different organisations, an agreement was reached.

THE WHOLE IS GREATER THAN THE SUM OF ITS PARTS

Whilst each representative could clearly articulate how his or her specific professional interest could contribute to the service, the ongoing discussions not only enabled each party to better understand the perspective of the others, but also to enrich the understanding of the critical and core debates around their own professional input.

The very process of debate in the quest for a common position cemented an understanding, which continues to flourish years later. Whilst this debate was between representatives of large national organisations, the opportunities abound for nurses, clinicians and social services staff in their day-to-day working to achieve the same synergy. The learning from being engaged in the process can be immense, and learning together is so often a means of cementing enduring professional relationships.

Working together

THE MESSAGE IS MORE EFFECTIVE IF THE MESSENGERS OWN AND PROMOTE IT

The message in this case was encapsulated in two products, two joint statements on the care of older people. Initially, the target audiences were the respective professional groups represented by the membership of the British Geriatric Society, the Royal College of Nursing and the Association of Directors of Social Services. However, as the debate within the associations grew, and documents began to be shared with wider social policy audiences, the effectiveness and ownership of the message developed between the partners. As each group shared information about the initiative within their own associations, the real strengths of the joint position began to emerge.

HOW COMPETITION CAN DELIVER POLICY AS WELL AS PRACTICE CHANGE

Somewhat to the surprise of everyone, we received an invitation to present jointly evidence to the Parliamentary Health Committee on the issue of continuing care. It was clear that, within the context of the national debate, to examine the implications of conflicts of interest within the system of continuing care and to achieve a joint agreement had a potency that none of us had recognised. A document that initially was intended to inform our professional colleagues of better forms of practice began to shape the national debate on continuing care and thus made a contribution to strategic policy formation.

Chapter **Eleven**

Fundraising for health care

Christa Paxton

OVERVIEW

Most people are involved with fundraising in some way or another either in their work or in their private life. The extent of this involvement might be at a relatively low level, for example buying a flag from a charity on a Saturday morning, or might entail full involvement as a member of a fundraising committee. There is a number of political debates about the use of voluntary funding in the NHS, but these are outside the scope and focus of this book. This chapter provides a general overview of the issues linked with fundraising, rather than entering into a philosophical or political debate.

THE ROLE OF FUNDRAISING WITHIN THE NHS

Historically, charitable funding had a role to play in health care but the introduction of the NHS in 1948 meant that non-statutory, voluntary funding sources became less important. Ever since the NHS was founded, charitable monies have been raised and spent on a variety of care, research and comfort needs that were not considered priority or significant in overall funding terms – the welfare needs of patients and staff, medical research and those care items that make a hospital stay more comfortable. In recent years, however, this charitable funding has grown extensively.

The 1980 Health Services Act allowed health organisations to raise monies directly from the public for the first time since 1948 and it also allowed Health Authorities to use some of their non-voluntary monies to initiate charitable appeals

With the NHS and Community Care Act of 1990 came the discontinuation of all of the established NHS funding arrangements and the introduction of the contract culture, with its purchasers and providers. NHS Trust boards now had to consider the potential conflict between their financial duties, which are to break even and earn a 6% return on capital whilst staying within the external financial limits (EFLs) set by the secretary of state, all within the context of this new contract culture.

It was this NHS and Community Care Act that led to the huge growth in the number of NHS bodies empowered to hold charitable funds. The 1996 statistics from the Charity Commission identified 25 000 charities within the National Health Service (entitling them to full exemption from corporation tax, income tax, capital gains and business rate discounts) and 2318 independent appeals within NHS establishments registered with the Commission. However during 1997 the Charity Commission updated its Register of Charities, became fully computerised and undertook a review of all NHS charities within England and Wales – that is, all those which are administered by health service bodies.

A process of rationalisation took place and is currently ongoing as a result of this review and 1998 figures available from the Charity Commission show 535 umbrella charities and 3207 subsidiary/special purpose charities. The Charity Commission agreed an arrangement whereby health service bodies operating more than one distinct charity would register one main charity – the umbrella charity with wide objects. Those charities with narrower objects operated by the same health service body would be registered as subsidiaries.

Income from all voluntary sources within NHS establishments and health service bodies has grown dramatically over the last two decades. The 1996/97 Department of Health figures for England alone show that total NHS charitable donations reached £141 million. This does not include the rest of the UK or any monies from investments which would make the total charitable income figure a good deal higher. One must then consider the impact of charitable medical research funding in the UK, some of which will cross-reference with the NHS charitable income figures. The Association of Medical Research Charities represents 99 registered charities which have as their principal activity the support of medical research in the UK. The AMRC figures for 1996/97 estimate that approximately £420 million is spent on medical research in the UK, with 48% of this figure being accounted for by the Wellcome Trust alone.

More charitable or voluntary monies than ever are being raised for capital building projects, basic core services, medical research in the form of project funding, units, named departments and research supported by some charities' own institutes. There has been a huge rise in equipment donated as a result of specific appeals, most notably in relation to those areas of health care which reflect the public's priorities and often offering emotional appeal – cancer, heart disease, hospices, neonatal and paediatric care. For example, most, but not all scanners, are funded from charitable appeals. BLISS, the national charity for newborn babies raises monies specifically to provide neonatal equipment to NHS hospitals for the care of premature and at-risk newborn babies, and funds specialist training for nurses and helpline support for parents.

From April 1997, for the first time, holders of NHS charitable funds were required to submit annual returns to the Charity Commission showing the true extent of charitable funding. This will also allow research to determine whether or not there is a relationship between a high percentage of charitable income and other circumstances, for example a high profile, an emotive cause, a sound fundraising proposition or a high proportion of private patient income.

Fundraising for health care

RELEVANT FUNDRAISING OUTSIDE THE NHS

At the end of February 1998, the number of registered charities in the UK was 187 000. If you compare this figure with that of 41 000 in 1986, the overall growth in the not-for-profit sector becomes clear. A large proportion of the 187 000 charities are community groups, clubs, places of worship, sports and social clubs, schools and universities, trade unions, professional associations and included within this number are those charities already mentioned which operate within the NHS establishments. Approximately 4000 new charities are registered every year, and some merge or cease to be charities.

To put the issue in perspective, recent estimates by the Charities Aid Foundation of the overall income for the sector vary between £8.4 billion and £29.5 billion, with the top 500 charities in the UK in income terms contributing £4.4 billion. Thus it can be seen that of the 187 000 charities, some are extremely small in income terms. Indeed, in 1995, research at Aston Business School revealed that 89% of charities had an income of less than £100 000 per annum.

The UK has an extremely long tradition of charitable activity and charitable giving dating from before historically endowed funds such as the newly renamed Bridge House Estates Trust Fund, the thirteenth century-established Bethlem Royal Hospital and the Order of St. John.

The Charities Act of 1993 has brought in legislation and recommendations to strengthen accountability to reflect the size and the growth of the sector.

The nature of fundraising in the UK as the new millennium begins is very diverse. This chapter outlines broadly the main types of fundraising activities relevant to health care today (Box 11.1), and those less relevant are mentioned briefly.

Box 11.1   Main types of fundraising relevant to health care

- Fundraising from:
  Corporate and trust sources
  Individual donor sources
  Statutory sources
- Fundraising from the European Union
- Fundraising from press and PR-related sources
- Trading

The added value of collaboration

FUNDRAISING FROM CORPORATE AND TRUST SOURCES

This will include:

- corporate, trust and livery company donations,
- community trusts and foundations,
- corporate sponsorships,
- corporate promotions,
- cause-related marketing,
- capital appeals,
- gifts in kind, and
- secondments.

How to go about fundraising

Information about fundraising from trusts, foundations or a company's community budgets can be accessed by investigating the specific charitable-giving policy and finding out who administers it. It is possible then to obtain the criteria for accessing funds, which may change from year to year. If there is a match between the charity's criteria and your need, a proposal must then be submitted, within defined guidelines. The contents of a typical proposal are given in Box 11.2.

Box 11.2   A typical proposal

One page A4 covering letter
Annual report of your organisation
Two sheets A4 proposal + budget, covering:

- brief background to charity/organisational objectives, e.g. how long it has been established, significant accomplishments
- specific details about what the money is for – outline/timetable and budget
- mention any existing or past relationship with the trust or company if appropriate
- find some leverage – for example, the money could unlock or enable something else
- be explicit if you are asking for money for more than one year, and allow for inflation in your calculations
- if the project is ongoing, but not requesting money for more than one year, detail how you plan to fund the subsequent years
- if you are asking for part funding only, detail your other intended sources

---

Fundraising for health care

Larger amounts of corporate money will be obtained by approaching companies to consider a collaborative venture. This would normally be done by the business office of the organisation, rather than by one individual. This may take the form of cause-related marketing where a company enters into a relationship which is focused to raise money for a specific cause. For example, retailers such as WH Smith and Tesco have run 'equipment for schools' promotions.

Organisations may make corporate links with charities, and these relationships seek to offer added value to both parties. Such relationships may offer the opportunity of demonstrating:

- 'a warm glow',
- a commitment to helping to raise the profile of a major social issue,
- that the organisation is a caring employer and good corporate citizen,
- improved company brand and awareness,
- natural synergy,
- improved staff morale,
- improved local profile and links, demonstrated through press, PR and media coverage,
- measurable outcomes, specifically in terms of company image, and sales,
- coverage and awareness, or
- links with pioneering work.

Ethical considerations must always be taken into account to ensure that any such partnership does not damage either side's reputation in any way.

A discrete capital appeal for, typically, a building or sometimes major equipment, may be launched under the overall umbrella of corporate and trust fundraising. A good capital appeal would rely upon a lengthy lead-in time in order to undertake the planning and investigations necessary to produce a sound business plan (Box 11.3). A capital appeal will rely heavily on the ability to build and maintain relationships. An organisation with any form of alumni will have an advantage, particularly if the details are kept up to date on a good database and the alumni are likely to have some disposable funds or networks to offer.

There are two important areas to consider when planning a capital appeal:

1. Ensure that there is total commitment from the staff and volunteers before beginning a campaign. It is usual for

The added value of collaboration

> **Box 11.3**   A sound business plan
>
> - Background
> - Need
> - Table of gifts
> - Marketplace and competition
> - Methodology and who does what
> - Ways to approach different donors
> - Interface between the appeal, and the organisation/charity
> - One unifying theme, logo and strapline (a *strapline* is a memorable phrase which captures the organisational mission focus)
> - Budget details
> - Timetable

hospitals and research institutes to have a range of 'soft' monies which are accessed by individual researchers or unit teams. It could be very damaging to the appeal if there were internal competition for funds from the same donors.

2. It is vitally important to have a clear idea of how to access revenue requirements for ongoing overheads and specific areas of service delivery. This avoids the trap of funding a building without ensuring a supporting revenue stream. This applies also to raising capital for a piece of equipment: it is important to be clear about the source revenue to support staff and/or consumables related to the equipment.

FUNDRAISING FROM INDIVIDUAL DONOR SOURCES

This includes:

- direct marketing,
- telephone fundraising,
- covenants and tax efficient giving,
- in memoriam donations,
- legacies,
- raffles and lotteries,
- events,
- community initiatives, and
- national and local organisations.

309

Individual giving or donor development programmes usually involve some method of capturing the interest of the individual via direct marketing, community activities, events or even telemarketing (using the telephone to talk about your cause and asking for a donation). Donors may be recruited in many ways, including house-to-house collections, sponsored events and street collections. However, that commitment may not include giving to other appeals. For instance, people who pay for a ticket to a charity event may well be doing so because they enjoy whatever the event is, seeing the event as entertainment. They view the charity connection as added value but they would be unlikely to give to the charity again. Donor capture and development is an increasingly sophisticated arena and not to be entered into lightly unless potential audiences have been researched, analysed and tested thoroughly. There are statutory rules and regulations surrounding fundraising activities such as street collections and house-to-house collections, so always ensure that these legal issues are investigated.

Hospitals and hospices are high in the legacy league tables – it is easy to make the link between someone's charitable giving and the fact that they know about a particular hospital or hospice as a result of personal contact. What is sometimes more difficult to sell in these terms is a non-life threatening disease. The public's response to medical research funding is often driven by emotion and the more emotive life threatening diseases can attract more monies.

A legacy campaign will involve researching target audiences, often via a direct marketing programme. This is normally managed by the marketing office of the organisation.

Community fundraising initiatives involve individuals working together in fundraising activities. In much the same way as a mailing might capture the interest of some people taking part in a local event, collecting door-to-door or in the street or selling raffle tickets in the pub will attract others. The secret of community fundraising lies in finding out about those activities people enjoy, and will do anyway, and then finding a way of adding a charity dimension to it. If you like pub quizzes, you will join in regularly and the skilful local fundraiser will use the opportunity to ask that the profits go to the local day centre, hospice, etc.

Any fundraising events should be part of a long-term planning process so that sufficient time is allowed to ensure that sponsorship is obtained, thereby maximising income. Before

The added value of collaboration

> **Box 11.4** Fundraising event: a checklist of issues to be considered
>
> - How much time, support and expertise are available?
> - How does the timetable look with reference to other local activities?
> - What are the legal implications and permissions?
> - Is registration with the local authorities and the police required?
> - What is your ability to sell the tickets?
> - Is any insurance needed?
> - Are licences necessary, i.e. if selling alcohol?
> - What press and publicity is required or available?
> - Would celebrity involvement be appropriate?
> - Is any sponsorship available?
> - What are the health and safety implications?
> - You will also need to prepare a detailed budget, including a contingency for unforeseen costs, costing in volunteer time and ensuring that cost:income ratios are identifiable (30:70 cost:income is a minimum guideline).

deciding upon any fundraising event the issues in Box 11.4 should be considered.

Any events which at the planning stage seem not to be cost-effective in terms of income/expenditure ratios should only be undertaken if your organisation has made a policy decision to do something for profile, the publicity value or the social and community value. Again, in the NHS and other health care organisations large events are normally managed centrally.

Use celebrities wherever possible by inviting them to participate, thereby endorsing the event. Continue to foster long-term relationships with public figures for future occasions. Sponsorship will make a huge difference as it enables costs to be covered. Local businesses, community groupings and trusts may be approached in the same way as outlined earlier when we discussed corporate fundraising. Use voluntary help to provide every possible assistance in terms of fact finding and preparation of proposals, always cross-referencing activities to avoid duplication of approaches.

Harnessing the skills of a good volunteer force is the key to moving into community activities. Good examples of this are hospital shops or the WRVS meals-on-wheels schemes. National organisations and their local groups may ensure a ready made volunteer force as well as funds. Approaches to Rotary clubs, Soroptimists, churches, sports and social clubs in the area, with a proposal or an offer to speak about the cause will often be a good starting point for promoting the organisation.

Raffles and prize draws using donated prizes are always popular. Giving with incentive has good results across charities, particularly if the prizes are good. Whilst donors recruited by this method do not always give because of the cause, they will often continue to respond to other incentivised offers. It is important to check the Gaming Board regulations before considering anything larger than selling tickets for a raffle as part of an event.

FUNDRAISING FROM STATUTORY SOURCES

Statutory sources of income are dealt with in Chapter 6. However increasingly, collaborative partnerships between the Department of Health, NHS organisations, academic institutions, local authorities and organisations such as the Health Education Authority are able to access funding for specific purposes. This is often linked with current government initiatives and more detail on collaborative fundraising is given later in this chapter.

FUNDRAISING FROM THE EU

The criteria to access EU funding require the organisation to be able to demonstrate that:

- the project requiring funding is transnational,
- pilot projects have been undertaken with good evaluated results,
- the project shows a multiplier/replicator effect,
- the project is innovative, and
- EU funding will not replace national funding.

Thus some longer term work stemming from a local health pilot project might well fit the criteria and allow the organisation to participate in a joint approach for funding of a larger, rolled-out project.

FUNDRAISING FROM PRESS AND PUBLIC RELATIONS (PR)-RELATED SOURCES

This includes:

- PR-related activities,
- patrons,
- press releases, articles and interviews,
- TV and radio appeals,
- advertising,
- events and exhibitions, and
- publications.

Any major fundraising must be well planned, particularly anything such as a local capital appeal. It is helpful to look for high-profile ambassadors for the cause and/or patrons who may bring contacts, networks, money, profile and influence to the appeal, whilst acting as figureheads within your organisation. Typically this may include all party political representation, celebrities who have a particular interest in the cause, writers, sportspeople and media names. Those who live or have connections locally are often keen to be involved with local appeals.

It is necessary to think about developing (sponsored if possible) newsletters, press packs, press releases and articles about the work and use these at every opportunity, distributing them to the supporters and national and local newspapers and magazines likely to be read by the target audience. Keep the relevant regional and national press corps members across all the media fully up to date with activities in such a way that they feel able to use your stories regularly. Media techniques are specialised skills, and all large organisations have individuals appropriately trained.

Develop items about fundraising activities and events at least 1–2 months in advance, longer if possible, to use in local magazines, and have several smaller pieces ready as 'remnant' space fillers. Some newspapers will offer a last minute space which they have not succeeded in filling with paid advertising. Local newspapers, particularly the free ones, are always looking out for stories and these could bring the fundraising a much needed profile. Similarly check to see if the appeal is likely to fit the criteria for both national and local television and radio charitable appeal slots.

Ensure that the appeal logo is used in all communications with the press and public and that all publicity material includes information about how to give money. Include a telephone number and contact name in any article, broadcast, interview or press release.

Develop transportable display boards and leaflets for national and local events, conferences and exhibitions. Get these sponsored and use as travelling exhibitions within the locality, at libraries, in supermarkets or community centres – wherever the target audiences may visit.

Above all, do not forget that in an interactive world it is worth considering developing a website to inform and gather supporters.

FUNDRAISING FROM TRADING SOURCES

Trading, from selling a few mugs and t-shirts, to running a charity shop in aid of your cause, has legislation of its own to consider. There are tax implications, but most importantly the charitable status of the appeal must be protected by adhering to the rules. The following points should be considered.

- The tax position
- Charity versus trading subsidiary
- Premises (if a shop)
- Competition in the marketplace
- Staffing and volunteers
- Stock and stock control
- Pricing.

Develop a marketing plan whatever the size of the operation. Remember to cost in all of the time elements. It often comes as a surprise to organisations setting out to sell goods in support of their cause, even on a small scale, to discover that processing orders, dealing with queries relating to orders, exchanging items, as well as developing stock control systems, takes a large amount of time. Always remember that the competition is run professionally and managed with the financial 'bottom line' always in mind.

If the hospital, hospice or appeal has a good enough brand and you intend producing trading items, you should ensure that you register the logo and trademark for future licensing purposes, which then could bring in further income. It is

The added value of collaboration

relatively cheap to do this and it protects the brand and gives greater bargaining power when it comes to entering a corporate promotion or sponsorship deal.

COLLABORATIVE PARTNERSHIPS WITH CHARITIES AND SPECIAL PROJECT FUNDING

A number of charities have traditionally worked in complementary ways with the NHS, notably St John Ambulance which is part of the ancient Order of St John, the British Red Cross and the Hospice Movement. For instance, 1995 figures show that 208 hospices provided beds and that 75% of these were funded by voluntary charitable income. Another example is the WRVS who bid for and win contracts within the NHS to provide services such as catering and shops in addition to their other mainstream voluntary activities.

It is quite common to find collaboration between NHS Trusts, local Health Authorities and an external funder for a specific piece of research or to establish a particular service from which all parties might benefit. Funding is usually secured on the basis of being able to find matching monies from the other parties. This can be complicated. The advantages for the project could include spreading the base of the funding to make the project more financially secure in the longer term. The disadvantages are linked to the public's reluctance to give money to replace what they see as the duty of government. As the NHS is seen as the role of government and the responsibility of the state, some people are uncomfortable with linking it with charities.

Some examples of collaborative ventures in the UK are outlined in Box 11.5.

Special project funding can be sought from a variety of sources, depending on the nature of the project. These might include:

- The Department of Health offering, for instance, Section 64 funding where the criteria for applications include 'innovative proposals of national significance that will complement statutory services and so help secure the provision of high quality health and social care for those who need it' (Department of Health Grants Administrations Unit 1997).

Fundraising for health care

The added value of collaboration

> **Box 11.5** Collaborative ventures: some examples
>
> - The Marie Curie Nursing Service is funded by a mix of charitable fundraising and NHS contracts.
> - The Director of Research and Development for the South and West regional office of the NHS Executive, responsible for commissioning the national R & D programme, has contracted the day-to-day management of its asthma research programme to the National Asthma Campaign.
> - Breakthrough Breast Cancer uses its charitable funds in support of its mission to fight breast cancer through research. In collaboration with the Institute of Cancer Research, the first specialist centre wholly dedicated to breast cancer research in the UK has been planned and opened. The Institute of Cancer Research in turn collaborates with the Royal Marsden Hospital over clinical developments, putting the research centre at the heart of the largest cancer complex in Europe. This creates an environment encouraging the sharing of ideas and experiences between scientists from and funded by a range of different organisations.
> - Yellow Brick Road is the fundraising campaign name of The Children's Foundation, based in Newcastle, which is an alliance between Newcastle University's Department of Child Health, the region's hospitals, businesses and families. It is a registered charity which funds important medical research into children's life limiting and life threatening illnesses.
> - The Neil Cliffe Cancer Care Centre is in the grounds of Manchester's Wythenshawe Hospital and is funded partly by the local Health Authority, partly by charitable fundraising and partly by the Macmillan Cancer Relief Fund, which is a registered charity in its own right.

- Trusts and foundations with a specific brief relating to health care, health care research or health care-related issues such as parenting, special needs and childcare
- Corporates with health care-related marketing objectives, which could include pharmaceutical companies wishing to fund a medical research project for or with a mainstream charity. This may extend their own research parameters and increase their visibility and customer reach. A collaboration with a corporate might involve support in kind as well as financial commitment.
- Linked in to the above point and on a broader scale, the government's private finance initiative (PFI) allows NHS hospitals to form collaborative partnerships with private

sector companies. PFI arrangements have been discussed in Chapter 6.

● The National Lotteries Charities Board now runs one continuous round of grants and should be investigated for funding. The Association of Medical Research Charities has played a role in ensuring joint bids for funding for medical research but there are many criteria into which an organisation might fit. To find out about the current round of grants available from the National Lotteries Charities Board at any one time telephone 0345 919191.

● The New Opportunities Fund might be appropriate to your project. The government has identified £200 million to establish a network of healthy living centres by the year 2001 with further monies to follow for health-related projects.

After the inception of the NHS in 1948, it soon became apparent that demand for health care was going to outstrip resources. Since the 1980s, demand has risen extremely rapidly, as medical technology has become more sophisticated and consumer expectation has grown. Since the inception of the internal market, organisations have been able to use financial resources in a more flexible way, which opened up the opportunities for charitable funding to occupy a higher profile in health care organisations.

CONCLUSIONS

This chapter has introduced you to fundraising as a coordinated and professional activity. Clearly, some organisations will use this funding source more than others, because of a range of differences such as size and core business of the organisation. It is important in all cases that any fundraising activity is carried out in a business-like and coordinated way in order that probity and accountability is ensured, and thus the confidence of the public is respected and maintained.

Fundraising for health care

Application 11:1 *Christa Paxton*

Resources for fundraising

Application 11.1 provides a directory of useful information about fundraising.

USEFUL ORGANISATIONS

It is useful to be able to access organisations that have up-to-date information about fundraising opportunities.

The Directory of Social Change

The Directory of Social Change runs courses and has very useful publications. They can be located at: 24 Stephenson Way, London NW1 2DP. Telephone: 020 7209 4949 (training courses), 0151 708 0117 (regional training courses), 020 7209 5151 (publications). Fax: 020 7209 5049. e-mail: info@d-s-c.demon.co.uk. Their publications include:

- *A Guide to UK Company Giving*
- *A Guide to Major Trusts*, which comes in two volumes
- *The CD ROM Trusts Guide – Funder Finder*
- *A Guide to Local Trusts*, with three volumes covering currently the North of England, the South and the Midlands
- *Organising Local Events*.

The Directory of Social Change also produces two magazines which are useful in fund-raising from trusts,

The added value of collaboration

318

foundations and companies. These are: *Corporate Citizen* and *Trust Monitor.*

The Charities Aid Foundation

The Charities Aid Foundation produce publications via Biblios Publishers' Distribution Services Limited. Their telephone number is: 01403 710851. The publications include the following:

- *Dimensions of the Voluntary Sector*
- *Grantseeker CD Rom*
- *The Directory of Grant making Trusts*, in three volumes.

The National Council for Voluntary Organisations

The NCVO runs courses, a consultancy service for smaller organisations and produces publications, and is based at: Regent's Wharf, 8 All Saints Street, London N1 9RL. Telephone: 020 7713 6161. Fax: 020 7713 6300. e-mail: 106007.1315@compuserve.com. Internet: http://www.vois.co.uk/ncvo.

The Institute of Charity Fund-raising Managers

Fundraisers within the UK have a trade body knows as the Institute of Charity Fund-raising Managers, which has regional groups and runs training and an accreditation scheme, as well as providing information on recommended fund-raising consultants. Their address is: 1 Market Towers, 1 Nine Elms Lane, London SW8 5NQ. For membership and enquiries about regional groups in East Anglia, London, the Midlands, Northern Ireland, the Northeast, the Northwest, Scotland, the Southeast, the Southwest, Wales and Yorkshire, contact: Telephone: 020 7627 3456. Fax: 020 7930 0687. *Business in the Community* and *Scottish Business in the Community* are useful publications when investigating community and corporate interest in your cause.

Resources for fundraising

Six Steps to **Effective Management**

The Charity Commission

The Charity Commission is available for advice. The three centres in England are London, Taunton and Liverpool and the telephone number for all three centres is 0870 333 0123. Their Internet address is: http://www.charity-commission.gov.uk.

SOURCES OF INFORMATION

Information about national and international companies

- *The Financial Times*/financial pages of all newspapers, *Financial Weekly* and the *Guardian*, amongst others, have profiles of key players within companies who have community initiatives
- Company annual reports
- *Beckett's Directory of City of London*
- *Stock Exchange Official Year Book*
- *Hambros Guide*
- *Guide to Key British Enterprises*
- *Who owns Whom*
- *Who's Who/Who's Who in the City*
- *Times 1000*
- *Kompass Register of British Industry and Commerce*
- *Jordan's Top Privately Owned Companies*
- *The Corporate Register.*

Information about local companies

- Local newspapers – financial pages and profiles
- Advertisements in local newspapers and magazines
- Chambers of commerce
- CBI Register of Contacts
- Kompass Regional Sections.

Most of these can be accessed through the public library.

Fundraising consultancies

AFC – The Association of Fund-raising Consultants: 01582 762446

ICFM – The Institute for Fund-raising Managers: 020 7627 3436

NCVO – The National Council for Voluntary Organisations: 020 7713 6161

Wolverhampton Coronary Aftercare Support Group

The Wolverhampton Coronary Aftercare Support Group (Registered Charity No. 701667) represents a model of good practice and partnership between the hospital and a group of volunteers. This case study outlines how it was set up, and how it has contributed to the quality of care for this group of patients.

During 1985 it increasingly became apparent that people in Wolverhampton who had suffered a heart attack were in need of further support and advice about their condition following discharge from hospital. Daily, the ward received telephone calls from previous patients enquiring about what they could and could not do. The anxiety experienced by both the patient and their family made it difficult for them to be clear about all the information shared with them in hospital. Very little concise written advice was available and any subsequent problems or worries were dealt with by their busy general practitioner.

There was a clear need to set up a help group to get together patients who had experienced general heart-related problems so that advice and guidance could be available to support them in returning to as normal a lifestyle as possible. Weekly evening meetings were organised to discuss health education topics. Patients and their families were encouraged to attend and participate at each session.

The added value of collaboration

By October 1986 the Wolverhampton Coronary Aftercare Support Group was well established with the help of a dedicated voluntary management committee composed mainly of previous patients of the Coronary Care Unit. Many founder members of this group are still active as committee members today. The aim of the group was to provide rehabilitation and exercise services for patients in Wolverhampton who have coronary artery disease. Funding for this service is provided by the group working in close cooperation with the Coronary Care Unit at New Cross Hospital and in collaboration with the Wolverhampton Health Authority.

The Group has a service level agreement with the Health Authority that totals £11 000 per annum. The remaining £50 000 required each year has to be raised by fundraising events and activities during the year such as an annual raffle, a garden party, fun walks, golf tournaments and steam railway outings. These are well supported and provide large contributions to the total amount required to maintain the agreed level of service. Other smaller events bring in more valuable financial support, along with considerable donations from various sources.

Most fundraising events are organised by the 25 strong committee and a number of willing helpers. The rehabilitation team generates some income by providing health care seminars to statutory and private organisations. Since the foundation of the group, in excess of £250 000 has been raised to be used within the Trust for the benefit of patients.

In consultation with the hospital authorities, a project was agreed to improve the access to the acute area of the coronary care unit, thus speeding up the admission time for patients following a heart attack. In addition a refurbishment of the area was agreed to install a 'state of the art' cardiac monitoring system capable of giving in-depth technical information about the cardiac patients. It was agreed also that sophisticated automatic emergency defibrillators would be installed at various points around the Trust site. This required a total of £150 000 and so the 'Have a Heart Appeal' was launched in October 1997 by the then Chancellor of the Exchequer, the Right Honourable Kenneth Clark QC, MP. Letters were sent to various contacts throughout Wolverhampton asking for support, and the local newspaper published weekly articles. The response

Wolverhampton Coronary Aftercare Support Group

was astounding and soon replies were flowing in offering financial support from many areas.

In February 1998 the new entrance and assessment suite was officially opened by Sir Jack Hayward OBE. The target had been achieved.

The group aims to supplement and complement the work of the hospital with an ever-increasing range of facilities and sees this as ongoing for as long as funds can be attracted. Many of the committed voluntary members are previous patients or relatives, who, out of gratitude for care and attention received, give their time willingly to assist with fundraising. This membership is expanding continually as more recent users of the service attend the group meetings. Their motivation is the desire to help 'give back a little' to benefit those similarly afflicted. Relationships are mutually beneficial. Funding is released by the group for appropriate staff to be appointed into Trust cardiac rehabilitation posts. The Public Relations Department in the Trust assists the group to gain publicity, and helps it to raise its profile in the community.

As a registered charity, the group has a management committee, and its own constitution. For joint ventures, appropriate officials come together to plan and manage the project, creating a successful alliance between the Royal Wolverhampton Hospitals NHS Trust and the Wolverhampton Coronary Aftercare Support Group. The joint efforts are highly successful in combining statutory funding with charitable funds to provide a 'gilt-edged service' for cardiac patients in Wolverhampton.

The added value of collaboration

Glossary

Glossary

Accruals Costs which have arisen, but for which an invoice has not been received. This often relates to items which accumulate over a period of time, such as electricity or water bills.

Adversarial relationship This arises where the two sides – supplier and customer – seek to gain at the other's expense. Some commentators say this occurred as a result of the internal market. The more collaborative approach of 'the new NHS' seeks to move towards partnerships. (See **Collaborative relationships**)

Annual budget Money allocated to a department or equivalent at the beginning of the year.

Apportioned overheads The proportion of general overheads that is attributable to a budget.

Asset Register Register of the capital resources within an organisation.

Audit trial To carry out activities and to maintain records in such a way that the processes are apparent and clear.

Block contract Under a block contract the purchaser pays a fee in return for guaranteed access to an agreed range of services.

Budget The financial expression of plans.

Budget holder Someone who has the authority, within specified conventions, to authorise expenditure.

Capital Expenditure on the acquisition of land and premises, individual works for the provision, adaptation, renewal, replacement and demolition of building: items or groups of equipment and vehicles etc.

Capital budget Money that is allocated to purchase items that have a life of more than one year, and items that cost (either individually or as a group) more than a specified figure.

Capital charges budgets Budgets kept to monitor that the level of capital charges (interest on capital and depreciation) matches that which was planned.

Capitation funding Method for allocating resources based on the principle of funding regions and subsequently districts to provide care for those living within their boundaries.

Glossary

Care Trusts Organisations in England, introduced by the NHS Plan, which combine Primary Care Trusts (i.e. NHS function) and local authority functions. They can therefore commission packages of client-centred services from one pot of money, which aims to achieve seamless service provision.

Case-mix costing Approach to costing which recognises that within speciality there can be a range of cases of different complexity and allows for differences between the more straightforward and the more complex cases.

Cash limit The amount of money the government proposes to authorise/spend on certain services or blocks of services in one financial year.

Clinical governance An initiative established to improve clinical standards at local level throughout the NHS. It requires clinicians to continuously improve quality, manage risk and safeguard standards and implement evidence based practice within a culture of partnership and collaboration.

Collaborative relationship A relationship where supplier and customer seek to work together to mutual benefit.

Commission for Health Improvement (CHI) A national statutory body established to provide independent scrutiny of local activity, particularly in relation to the quality of care. It has the power to intervene to address problems in organisations.

Community care Care, particularly for elderly people, people with learning or physical disabilities or a mental illness, provided outside a hospital setting, i.e. within the community.

Comprehensive spending review A review undertaken by the government looking into the spending within government departments such as health and education.

Contingency A sum of money included in the costing of a business case to cater for any unplanned and/or unpredictable expense during the project. This sum is not intended to support a change in specification.

Cost The measure of the value of resources lost as they are used or consumed by the organisation.

Cost-and-volume contract Under a cost-and-volume contract the purchaser buys a specific volume of service for a specified cost.

Cost-per-case contract Under a cost-per-case contract the purchaser agrees to pay a certain sum each time a particular activity takes place; generally used for more complex procedures.

Cost centre Department or equivalent for which a budget for expenditure on staff and material resources has been set.

Departmental budgeting Allocating resources to departmental cost centres under headings such as 'pharmacy', 'theatres', 'catering', etc.

Direct costs   Costs that can be directly attributed to the budget for a particular department, specialty or team.

Economy   Spending or consuming as little as possible, while still maintaining the required quality.

Education consortia   Groups of representatives from Trusts, Health Authorities and other organisations who deliver health care, e.g. the private sector, the prison service, etc. who have the responsibility for allocating resources for non-medical education and training (NMET) (i.e. education and training for all groups *except* doctors and dentists) for both pre- and post-registration activities.

Effectiveness   The use of resources to achieve the outcomes required.

Efficiency   Improving the relationship of resources input to outputs of workload accomplished.

Establishment   The level of staff allocated to a given area: this is usually described in WTEs (whole time equivalents).

External customer   Anyone who uses the service of the organisation, including both patients and clients (the end-users) and purchasing organisations.

Extra contractual referral (ECRs)   An arrangement within the internal market to enable a patient to receive treatment, via a referral, in a NHS Trust where no contract exists with the patient's Health Authority of residence or GP fundholder. These are being superseded by service agreements between Primary Care Groups/Primary Care Trusts or equivalent, and the providers of services, e.g. the Trusts.

Family Health Services (FHS)   Services provided in the community through general practitioners, dentists, pharmacists and opticians, all of whom are independent contractors, i.e. are not *employed* by the NHS but work within the NHS via a contractual arrangement.

Financial envelope   The amount of money available for a given project or activity.

Fit for purpose   A service which does what is necessary to meet the designated outcome.

Fixed costs   Costs you pay whatever the level of activity – the costs of land and buildings and, to a large extent, equipment.

Flexing   Method for modifying a budget during the financial year if the actual level of activity differs from that which was originally anticipated.

General Medical Services (GMS)   Medical services provided for individuals by general medical practitioners.

General practitioner fundholder (GPFH)   Family doctor practices which chose to accept an agreed budget for part of the practice activity and to manage that budget themselves. The budget covered practice staff, hospital referrals, drug costs, community nursing services and management costs. It was a discretionary part of the Health Authorities' spending. Since April 1999, GPFH has been replaced by local commissioning arrangements, which vary within the four countries in the United Kingdom. GPFHs have been abolished as a result of The Health Act (1999).

Gross expenditure   The total expenditure on health services.

Health Act   Act of Parliment (passed in 1999) to abolish the internal market.

Health Action Zone (HAZ)   An initiative to bring together organisations within and beyond the NHS to develop and implement a locally agreed strategy for improving the health of local people.

Health Authority   A Health Authority is responsible, within the resources available, for identifying the health care needs of its resident population, and for securing through its contracts with providers, a package of hospital and community health services to reflect those needs. The Health Authority has a responsibility for ensuring satisfactory collaboration and joint planning with the local authority and other agencies. During the period of the internal market, Health Authorities acted as 'purchasers', but their role has evolved to that of commissioning services.

Health Boards   The Scottish equivalent of Health Authorities.

Health Improvement Programme (HImP)   An action programme to improve health and health care locally, led by the Health Authority. It will involve NHS Trusts, local commissioning groups and other primary care professionals, working in partnership with the local authority and other interested parties, e.g. voluntary groups.

Healthy Living Centres   National lottery-funded facilities to help tackle the health and social needs of deprived communities.

Indirect costs   Costs which cannot be attributed directly to a particular budget but usually are shared between them.

IM & T   Information management and technology. See NHS information strategy.

Income budgets   Match planned and actual income.

Incremental budgeting (or historic-based budgeting)   Approach to calculating a budget based on the budget for the previous year, but with minor adjustments to allow for price increases, pay awards and any changes in service.

Inputs   The resources required to carry out a particular activity.

Internal customers   Staff/unit who require a range of goods and services from another department in the organisation to enable them to provide their own service to others. For example a group of wards will need to have the services of the catering department to provide food for the patients.

Internal market   The process of competition between purchasers and providers established following the 1990 NHS and Community Care Act. The first 'wave' of NHS Trusts was established in April 1991.

Internal suppliers   The departments (e.g. catering) who provide goods and services to another department (e.g. wards).

Local Health Care Cooperatives   These have replaced GP fundholding in Scotland with effect from April 1999. Their role is to coordinate primary care, mental health and community hospital services.

Local Health Groups   These have replaced fundholding in Wales with effect from April 1999. They are based largely on local authority areas with the aim of enabling effective commissioning of local services. They involve all GPs and other relevant health professionals.

Marginal cost   The cost of the extra resources needed to do another activity from a given baseline, e.g. to make an additional visit or to fill an additional bed.

Medical and Dental Education Levy (MADEL)   The budget used to fund pre-qualification medical and dental education.

Non-pay budgets (sometimes called 'non-staff' budgets)   Budgets for resources other than staff salaries such as materials and overheads.

Non-pay expenditure   The amount spent on everything except staff pay.

Opportunity cost   If you use a particular resource in one way, you lose the opportunity to use it in another – this would be termed as a *lost opportunity cost*.

Outcomes   The aims and objectives that the organisation is seeking to achieve.

Outputs   Workload accomplished as a result of using resources.

Overheads   Costs of services which support the general running of the organisation but which cannot be related to the activity level of an individual department, e.g. cleaning of corridors etc.

Pay budgets (sometimes called 'staff' budgets)   Budgets covering staff salaries.

Pay expenditure   The amount spent on staff salaries.

PCG   Primary Care Group.

PCT   Primary Care Trust.

Probity   Carrying out activities with honesty and integrity.

Quality   Consistently getting things right to the standards required by your patients or your customers.

Glossary

Six Steps to **Effective Management**

Quality financial information   The right information, available at the right time and in the right format.

Rationing   Limiting the availability of a particular service, treatment or procedure, whether explicitly, via exclusions, or more implicitly, by clinical judgement and waiting lists.

Recharges   Charges made for services (like X-ray or physiotherapy) provided by other departments.

Recurring costs   Costs which recur, e.g. regular maintenance contracts, staff salaries. These should be taken into account when planning capital investment, e.g. purchasing of a large piece of equipment. Consideration must be given to whether or not the unit can afford to maintain and staff the facility once it has been purchased.

Reporting period   The period covered by the budget statement.

Revenue budgets   Revenue budgets allocate money for day-to-day running costs such as salaries, medical supplies, heating, lighting, drugs and other consumable materials.

Service level agreement (SLA)   An agreement between departments or directorates to provide a certain level of service at an agreed price; designed to ensure clear responsibility and control of internal budgeting.

Setting priorities   Deciding what you will put first – which services will be provided, and to whom.

Skill mix   The range and variety of skills held by members of a team or department. This is more usually translated into a mix of designated roles, e.g. 3 seniors, 4 juniors, etc.

Snoozelen   A word used to describe a room that is furnished and fit to provide a calm, soothing environment for patients/clients.

Stakeholders   Those people, groups of people or organisations who have a legitimate interest in the activity or project.

Standard   Measure against which performance can be monitored.

Start-up costs   Costs which are incurred as a result of a new project – sometimes referred to as *front loaded costs*.

Unit cost   The average cost of a unit of activity – in other words a diagnostic visit, test, bed day, operation, meal, etc. It is derived from establishing the cost of a service or function and dividing by the outputs of that service or function.

Value for money (VFM)   Term used in the NHS to embrace the three Es: economy, efficiency and effectiveness.

Variable costs   Costs that increase in relation to the level of activity – in particular, supplies.

Variance   The difference between planned and actual expenditure.

Virement   Transferring funds from one category of expenditure to another.

Glossary

Weighted capitation Process of allocating funding to districts based on number of people living within each district, adjusted for the age profile of the district, the relative social and economic circumstances of the population, and certain other factors such as the training of staff and regional factors including the extra cost of London.

Workforce Development Confederations Organisations which evolve from Education Consortia in 2001. They will have the responsibility of ensuring an appropriately skilled workforce to meet the health needs of their local population. They will be based alongside the local health authority.

WTE Whole-time-equivalent staff members.

YTD (year to date) This usually identifies the total amount that has been spent on a particular resource since the beginning of the financial year.

Zero-based budgeting Approach to calculating a budget that starts with a blank sheet of paper and requires managers to decide what they want to do, how much this will cost and to justify the desired level of expenditure.

Index

Six Steps to **Effective Management**

Index

Index

Index

Index

size of sector, 272
and winter admissions, 141
Nursing staff
breast care specialists, 279
private and NHS working, 279
workforce planning, 160–163

Older people
Care trusts, 43
continuing care, 86–91, 271–275, 292–299, 300–302
mental health services, 86–91
Operational planning, 102–103, 104, 112–113
Opportunities, SWOT analysis, 109–110
Opportunity costs, 233
Option appraisal exercise, 192–197, 236
Organisational change *see* NHS organisational structures; NHS reforms
Organisational culture
and personal development, 166
and quality of care, 85, 262–263
Organisations, definition, 6–7

Parliament, 37–38, 173
Partnership contracts, employer–employee, 146–147
Partnership working
budgetary monitoring, 206
charitable fundraising, 303–324
Community Health Councils, 275–277
in continuing care, 86–91, 271–275, 292–299, 300–302
and financial control, 185
mental health services, 86–91
NHS structures, 33, 34, 38–39, 43, 57, 58–63, 67, 73–74
private finance initiative, 183–184, 316–317
voluntary agencies, 280–287, 300–302, 311–312
workplace learning, 148, 287–290
Pay, budgetary controls, 208
People, theory of, 262
Performance data reviews, 129–131
Performance indicators, 206, 233–234
Performance management, 99–100

Performance monitoring, 82–85, 128–129
'earned autonomy', 40
Personal development, 84, 145, 146, 147–149, 161, 164–169
see also Education and training
Personal development plans (PDPs), 161, 166–169
PEST analysis, 108–109, 110
Planning *see* Business planning
Political agendas
business planning, 98–99
financial management, 177
NHS structures, 31–35, 36–38, 64–66
quality improvement, 250
Political (PEST) analysis, 108
Portugal, health care system, 11–12
PR-related fundraising, 313–314, 323–324
Pre-Operative Assessment Clinic (PAC), 192–197
Press-related fundraising, 313–314, 323–324
Primary Care Groups (PCGs), 24, 38–39, 46, 48, 49–56
and CHI, 55
mental health for older people, 87–89, 90
and resource allocation, 180–181
Primary Care Trusts (PCTs), 45, 48, 49–56
and resource allocation, 180–181
with social services (Care trusts), 43, 52
Primary data sources, 110, 111
Private finance initiative (PFI), 183–184, 316–317
Private health sector *see* Independent sector
Private/public sector interdependence, 98
Prize draws, 312
Professional accountability
clinical governance, 41–42, 53, 82–83, 251–252
as driver of NHS reform, 15
Professional development *see* Education and training
Profound knowledge, 262
Project management, 103, 104
Prospective payment system (PPS), 29, 30–31

Index

Index

Six Steps to **Effective Management**